Goodbye Cancer, Hello Health

Goodbye Cancer, Hello Health

What God Taught Me on My Own Journey

Donna Marie Hockley, NHC, MPCP

Raveonna Publishing
Cawston, British Columbia V0X 1C1

Goodbye Cancer, Hello Health

ISBN:978-1-9991745-4-5

Edited by Raveonna Publishing

Cover Photograph
taken by Emma Eichhorn
of her sister Kiara Eichhorn

Illustration picture drawn by
Melody Love Lindelauf

Author's Disclaimer

The following information is based upon the research, training and personal experience of Donna Marie Hockley. Unfortunately, I cannot be held responsible for the decisions that you may make after reading this book.

You have the right to consult other healthcare professionals (A Naturopath Doctor, Herbalist, Natural Health Consultant, Nutritionist, or a Medical Doctor) and you also have the legal and God-given right to treat yourself, but you must also assume the responsibility of doing so. Donna Marie and Raven Hockley of Health in Balance Educators are not doctors, and thus are not a substitute for other medical care that you may choose to seek.

Legally, this book can not contain any guarantee that you will have the same results that I, nor the testimonials of those you will read in this book had. But if after reading what I learned on my own journey with cancer, it makes logical sense to you, remember that it is your body and do not let anyone scare you into doing anything that you do not feel 100% convinced is going to move you towards restoring your health. Only YOU can make these choices.

May God bless you and guide you on your journey back to wellness.

Dedication

This book is dedicated to a few different people.

First of all, to my loving Father in heaven (God). You invite me to call You Abba, which simply means 'Daddy.' You kept me alive against all odds when I had Leukemia as a child, much to the amazement of the doctors. Then, when a chiropractor noticed the swelling in my lymph nodes back in 2005, and I was diagnosed a second time forty-two years later, with cancer, You directed me on what to do in order to get well. Without Your direction on how to help my body recover, I know that I would not have survived.

I want to thank my husband Raven for your unending love and support, when I chose to go strictly the natural route, against the protest of family and friends. I am so grateful that we were 'on the same page', and that I did not have the extra stress of feeling like I was all alone in my conviction that I wanted to do what God led me to do. I am also grateful for your encouragement when I felt a deep passion to write this book so that I could share what I had learned on my journey with cancer.

Next, I would like to dedicate this book to my children. I know that when I told you that I had been diagnosed with cancer, you were so scared that I would die. As a mother, my greatest fear is that if either of you ever developed cancer, that you might listen to 'the specialists' and go the medical route. May this and my previous book, be a blueprint of what will give you a much higher chance for full recovery (long term), if you ever find yourselves in that situation.

To my good friend Dorothy; I will be forever grateful for your unselfish support of taking my carrots home to wash and re-bag for me when I did not have the energy to do it for myself. Thank you, thank you, thank you.

To Julie, my step-daughter; I am grateful that out of my love for you and your dad, when we heard that they found a tumor on your brain, I became even more serious about completing this book. I knew that I wanted you to have this knowledge as quickly as I could write it. I am also grateful for the feedback and questions that you asked, to help me know what things I needed to include.

Last, but definitely not least, this book is dedicated to you the reader. I don't know your situation, but I know that you are reading this book for a reason. It may be for yourself, or to help someone you care deeply for. If it is to help someone, make sure to read the chapter called; 'Support, Support, Support'. If you are reading this book for yourself, may this book be exactly what you were hoping it would be, so that you can confidently make choices of what you would like to do on your healing journey.

Table of Contents

Section 1
From My Heart to Yours

A Personal Note to My Readers

Hi there!

Thank you for taking the time to read this book. I am so happy that you have chosen to educate yourself on the health principals that I personally have found assisted my body to come back into balance, when diagnosed with any 'dis-ease', including cancer.

If you have not read my first book; 'What You *NEED* to Know To Survive Cancer', and if you are at all questioning if chemo, radiation, surgery, or even a biopsy is your best option, then I want to encourage you to stop reading, and first read that book. You will absorb a lot more out of this one, if you are convinced that going 100% the natural route from this day forward, is <u>your</u> best option.

If you have already done chemotherapy, you need to know the critical facts that are discussed in the chapter called; 'But, I already did chemo!' of that same book. Unfortunately, not knowing about the ramifications of having Chemotherapy Resistant Cancer Cells, and what you can do about them, could mean the difference between surviving or not.

You can pick up a copy on one of my websites; **www.DonnaMarieHockley.com**, or **www.AreYouinBalance.com**. Another place that you can purchase them, is at a workshop that I am speaking at in your area. It is available as both a soft cover, as well as an e-book so as to help people obtain instant access to this critical information. At this point, in addition to the English version, the first book has also been translated into Spanish. My goal is to eventually have all of the books available in English as well as translated into Spanish.

If you are now ready to get started reading this book, I would like you to know that it was written to answer two questions that I am asked over and over again.

The first one is; "What did you do Donna?"

When people hear that I had cancer as a child, and then again back in 2005, (forty-two years later), and that I went 100% the natural route, they want to know what I did to regain my health.

I am hoping that by writing this book, it will provide an avenue for me to help save my husband from having to endure the wait time over and over again, as I describe what I did, when faced with this question. 😊

The second question I often get is; "Can I give your phone number to my friend/relative who has cancer". My answer has always been; "Absolutely!"

Unfortunately, reality is that very few people actually do call. As much as this loving person desires to help those that they care about, it is not achieving their goal.

Writing this book provides another way for people to pass along what I would tell their loved one, if we did have the opportunity to talk or even work together on their healing.

Of course, another option would be to gain the education through reading these two books, and then having the lifelong ability to share what you have learned, with family and friends.

Do you understand why I NEEDED to write this book?

So let's get started!

Introduction

Being told that "you have cancer", is one of the most life altering moments that you and I have experienced. For me, it altered my whole perspective of what is truly important to me. My life changed forever... for the good.

Unfortunately, when it is discovered that you have developed cancer, often the whirlwind of appointments very quickly begin, even before you have had time to digest the diagnosis.

I want to encourage you to stop, breathe and think clearly of what you truly want to do. It is YOUR body, and you are the ONLY ONE who can choose what you want to do, and what is not even an option. It is ok to say that you would like to take a few days to digest this news, before agreeing to go for any appointments.

Just because it was discovered that you have cancer today, does not mean that you need to "start treatment" tomorrow. What if they had not discovered it for another week or two? The chances are high that it would be no different than today. I personally saw the swelling in my lymph nodes for about a year before my chiropractor saw it. I thought I was just gaining weight and did not pay attention to it.

So please, do not let anyone, not your doctor, nor your family or friends, rush you into a decision based on fear. You do have time to make a rational, informed choice.

I am going to assume that you are reading this book because you have a desire to work on restoring your health. You want to move towards being in better health than before you even knew that you had developed cancer. I am sure that you want your energy to return too.

My desire for you, is to never have to worry about being surprised that your cancer has returned, nor having to endure losing all of your hair, or becoming best friends with your toilet.

If you follow all twelve health principals outlined in this book, your body will naturally be moving into the zone where cancer cannot survive. Of course, if you go back to doing things that set your body up for your immune system to go down, then your body will start to let you know, but at least you will have the blueprint to get back on track.

If you are a Christian, I want to encourage you to do what I did; to pray and ask God for direction. He will guide you on His methods.

If you are not a Christian, that is Ok, I believe that this book will give you the honest information that will help you make wise choices. Choices that can put you back into the driver's seat and increase your chance of survival.

I have had people think that they can do what I outline in this book, along with the medical route. To be very honest with you... I beg you, to reconsider that thought, for your own good. Go back and read my first book, as I truly believe with every ounce of my being, that you would be playing with fire, which will end up burning you... badly. As I hear testimonial after testimonial, I have seen that the results of that choice are rarely favorable for long term health.

If you have been told that you have stage two, three or four, or that it is aggressive, do not let that scare you into doing anything different than if you were told that the cancer is stage one, or slow growing. What this means is that it has spread from the original place where it first started.

What it also means, is that you need to be very serious about following ALL of the health principals that are discussed in the following chapters. You cannot afford to play with it.

Remember though that there are many people who have also had stage 2, 3 or 4, and have changed the environment that disease thrives in. They are well and extremely healthy today. How? Changing the reason that they developed cancer in the first place.

Chris Wark had stage three, and beat cancer by doing most of what I teach in this book. Veronica was only given two weeks to live, and she also beat cancer by following the health principals that rebuild the health. So, if you have been given more than two weeks to live, you are ahead of the game. 😊

If you are told that the cancer is aggressive, again do not buy into the fear. If they tell you that you only have a few months to live, consider what Veronica did. She immediately started working on rebuilding her immune system. She gave her body the tools that it needed in order to heal. She stopped doing the things that were feeding her cancer, and not only did she not die in the predicted two weeks, her body started to quickly heal. I strongly believe that destroying your immune system through what the medical system offers, is really counterproductive.

If you are feeling compelled that you are needing to stop the cancer quicker than you believe changing your inner environment will do, then I would encourage you to use a herb called Paw Paw. Unlike chemotherapy, it does not destroy your immune system, but instead cuts off the energy to the cancer cells, while leaving your healthy cells alone. It is the best alternative that I know of, compared to destroying your immune system by using chemotherapy. You can read more about it in Section 6 in the chapter called; 'What about Herbs and Supplements?'

The hard truth is, that if the cancer is moving at such an aggressive rate that the American Paw Paw cannot stop the cancer in its tracks, then nothing would have helped you, including chemotherapy. BUT... your chances of being in that situation, is VERY low. You have an excellent chance that you have enough time to turn this nightmare around. But you do need to be very serious.

You need to understand that Paw Paw will only destroy the cancer cells, so you also need to address the root cause of why you developed cancer in the first place, by working on rebuilding your immune system. It is a huge mistake to think that you can just take a single herb and be fine long-term. The health principals described in the upcoming chapters, will help you get back on track.

My sole motive for sharing this book with you, is that I want YOU to live.

I also want you to not be plagued with the constant fear of wondering "will it resurface it's ugly head again?" With what you are going to learn, you will have the tools to be in charge of your own health, now and forever.

If as you read, you find that you really would like support from a community of other people who are also following these principals, you may want to join the online program that I plan to offer. You will find more info in the final chapter of this book called; 'Where to Go from Here'.

So, are you ready to be able to exclaim from the roof tops; 'Goodbye Cancer, Hello Health'? Let's dive in and discover how to be loving to your body, rather than destroying your immune system!

Section 2
A Bird's Eye View

The Whole Enchilada

Whenever my husband and I travel to unfamiliar territory, we often look up the address on Google Map. We start with the satellite view. Then we move into looking at it from an aerial advantage. Lastly, we move down to street level so that we can get a much closer view of what is surrounding the address that we desire to arrive at.

In the case of your health, we will also start with the very broad view by using an acronym, which is like putting the address into Google Map. It tells you where you want to end up, but you need to look closer to see what it entails.

My intention behind creating an acronym, stemmed from my husband and I having the desire to help people to be able to remember each of the letters for two important reasons.

First of all, each letter represents one of the twelve health principals that I have found needs to be addressed in order to truly get well from ALL diseases, including cancer.

Cancer is just at the far end of the spectrum of disease. You cannot go any further downhill than cancer.

Please understand that this is not a buffet that you can pick and choose which ones you want, or think that you can do. Every one of them are important. You need the 'Whole Enchilada', in order to have all of the parts that it takes to regain your health.

Over the years, I have observed that many people only focus on one aspect of health, which is usually either what foods to eat, or what herbs to take. What you eat or don't eat is important, but it is only one of twelve aspects.

As a Natural Health Consultant, Counsellor, Christian, and a cancer survivor, I have come to grasp the full picture that we are a whole human being.

In order to get well and stay well long term, we need to address not just our physical, but also our emotional, mental and spiritual areas.

The second reason that I wanted both you and I, to be able to easily remember the twelve health principals, is to be able to quickly identify which area a person is currently out of balance.

When my chiropractor noticed a swelling back in 2005, I was already very health conscious. I ate pretty healthy, exercised daily, got lots of fresh air, and drank plenty of water. I didn't smoke, nor use any prescription or 'recreational' drugs and had not had any alcohol for years.

Upon going over this acronym, I was able to see that there were a couple of areas that I was not even thinking about. It helped me pinpoint what had contributed to my immune system going down. With that information, I was able to take the necessary steps, back towards health.

Does that make sense?

I am hoping that by me laying it all out for you, it will give you a 'Bird's Eye View' of the road that we will be taking together.

Let's start by looking at what this mysterious acronym is;

pH. D. A. N. S. W. E. R. S. A. B. C.

Any time I see a client who is unsure of what has led to their 'dis-ease', we go over these health principals to see which ones we need to work on, while continuing the others that they are already doing.

If you read my first book 'What You *NEED* to Know To Survive Cancer', I talked about the challenging task of looking to see what lifestyle habits have contributed towards you developing cancer. The next page is where you can start to discover your answer! ☺

I will provide you with the words associated with each letter of the acronym, which is like the Arial view. You may want to refer to the following page... often, as this is your Health Rebuilding Blueprint.

We will be going into a lot more detail on exactly what they each mean and how you incorporate them into your life on a daily basis, for long-term health. So here they are.

pH Balancing

Detoxification

Air

Nutrition

Sunshine

Water

Exercise

Rest and Relaxation

Stress Reduction

Attitude of Gratitude

Beyond yourself

Comical

In the next three sections, we will get down to street level, for you to be able to clearly see the whole picture. You will come away with knowing what to do to start implementing these health principals into your life…starting today!

So, let's get started on your healing journey.

Section 3
Getting Your
pH D

Life Is in the Balance

Are you getting your 'pH.D'?

What do I mean when I ask if you are getting your 'pH.D'? Do you need to go to university to get it?

No, your 'pH.D'. stands for the two most critical foundations that the last ten health principals build upon. Both of these two components work hand in hand to create an environment that cancer cannot survive in. This is our goal isn't it!?

So, if the acronym 'pH.D', has nothing to do with going to university, what does it stand for?

The pH part stands for Potential for Hydrogen. Don't worry what that means, as understanding what a potential for hydrogen is, will not get you well. Doing things that will bring your body into balance, is what is important. In the meantime, let me see if I can keep this as simple as possible.

The whole purpose of writing this book is to help you understand how to change the environment of your body, so as to not be a good host to diseases, and especially cancer.

So why is pH balancing so important? Do you remember in my first book, the example about mold only growing in a dark, damp environment? Well cancer also will only grow in certain environments.

For eighteen months I had been following to the best of my ability most of the health principals that you will read in section four and some of the ones in section five. I wasn't doing it perfect, but the best that I could at the time. (In my own strength of course.)

During those eighteen months, my tumor marker didn't get worse, which was great, but it also did not get better. ☹

I prayed and asked God to show me that what I was doing was helping. His answer to me was; "My grace is sufficient for you".

Two weeks later, a friend brought to my attention about pH balancing. I knew with every ounce of my being, that this was a critical component that I had missed. This led me to research even more about pH balancing, as well as the 'D' part that makes up the last part of pH.D., came onto my radar.

Even though, as a Natural Health Consultant I was aware of both of them, I had not placed the importance on them. Sometimes, our answers are right in front of us, but unfortunately, we do not see them. This is when an outside source can be exactly what we need at that point on our journey.

Unfortunately, I have discovered that like myself, very few people realize of how critical these two components are, but I am no longer making that same mistake.

When I implemented these two health principals into the rest of the program, in just six short weeks, for the first time in almost two years, my tumor marker dropped in half!

In this chapter I will first teach you what pH is, and why it is so important. Then we will look at how you test it, and of course, the most important part; how do you achieve it?

I will be referring to a pH chart throughout this section. Originally, I had it included... right here! Unfortunately, when I discovered that most e-readers do not show the color in the pictures, and that having even one page with color on it, jumped the printing price way up, I had to rethink this. So, what I have done, is I have posted the chart on my website **www.AreYouinBalance.com.** I know that it is not the best solution, but I wanted you to have this book while I searched for another option.

Do you have the chart in front of you? You will notice a couple of things. First you will notice that on the far left, the color is yellow, on the far right it is purple and smack in the middle, it is green. When you test your pH, the special litmus paper will show a color somewhere from yellow to purple. The goal is to have it show dark green, which is the color of nature. No need to worry about memorizing the colors on this chart, as when you purchase your own testing strips, it comes with a similar chart.

You will also notice that the chart only shows from 5.5 – 8.0, but in actuality the numbers go from 0 – 14. Your goal is to have your pH be consistently between 6.8 and 7.2 as that is where optimum health is. Perfect health is at 7. (God's favorite number)

From 6.8 down to 5.8, this is the environment where all diseases set up in the body.

Below 5.8 is where cancer thrives. It doesn't mean you have cancer. It just means that the environment is ripe for it. Most North Americans are at 5.2, which is why I believe that cancer is going through the roof.

They say that cancer is the second leading cause of death, behind heart disease, and according to the July 2000 issue of the Journal of the American Medical Association, the third leading cause of death, is prescription drugs.

Recently when I was reading our local paper, I was witnessing in the obituaries, almost every single person who recently died, had 'lost the battle to cancer'. I was wondering if cancer had now surpassed heart disease and had moved into the top leading cause of death. When I read the Canadian 2018 statistics, I saw that yes cancer had just moved into first place here in Canada. ☹

Back to learning more about how important pH is!

Testing your pH is one of the most accurate ways to know how healthy you truly are. When I first tested myself, my pH was not even registering on the test strips which means that it was below 5.5

Our bodily fluids (blood, urine, salvia, lymph), all can tell us so much of what is truly going on inside of our bodies. But before you run to your doctor asking for them to test your blood pH, let me explain why they will think that is a pretty silly request.

Our bodies were created to keep us alive for as long as it can. The pH of our blood needs to be kept in a very tight range of between 7.35 and 7.45. If our blood pH drops lower or goes higher than this, you actually could die, so our blood does everything it can to maintain this tight spectrum.

How does it do that? Like Robin Hood, the blood will steal from the body, minerals to bring it back into balance. Minerals are a key element that our bodies need to operate properly. In fact, they are more important than vitamins. When we don't have enough magnesium, we start to get heart palpitations. When we don't have enough calcium, we develop soft bones and teeth. Without enough sodium and potassium, our electrolyte balance goes all crazy and a lot of different symptoms occur from that.

So now that you know that the body needs minerals and will rob them in order to keep you alive, what might be a key component for foods to be rich in?

If you guessed minerals, you are absolutely right! If you guessed something different, or you were stumped, that is ok, your secret is safe with me.

But before we get into what foods and beverages I am referring to when I say 'pH balanced', it is important to find out where you are starting from, and then you will know where you need to get to.

So how do you test your pH?

Here is how you test yourself in the privacy of your own home;

Get pH test strips from a health food store in their supplement section, or you can order them off of my website. It is important to find pH test strips that look similar to the chart that I described a few pages back, and that you saw on my website. We don't want you getting ones that are meant for testing your swimming pool. You also want to have the twelve increments from 5.5 – 8.0, so as to test more accurately where your pH currently is.

You've got your test strips? Great! Now, take a sample of your urine 1st thing in the morning (the 1st urine after 2 am), before you eat or drink anything. The best way to do this is to use a small, paper 'Dixie' type cup and catch a sample of your urine in it.

Dip a strip of the litmus paper into your urine and shake off any excess. Do not just 'pee onto the paper', as it will not be accurate due to the force hitting the paper.

Immediately match it to the color coding on the package. Write down what the number is. Repeat this for at least 4 days in a row, then you will know the numbers that you are starting with.

Below 6.8 is called acidic. Between 6.8 and 7.2 is called Alkaline Balanced. Above 7.2 is an over alkaline, which really is also acidic and not where health is.

I had a friend who after hearing about pH balancing in a workshop I facilitated, checked her husband's pH and called to tell me that she was so happy because it was almost 8. I explained that no, this was too high. A few weeks later he had a major stroke. So, remember, more is not better when it comes to your pH.

Now what?

Now that you know where you are starting from, I will wager a bet that your pH was not between 6.8 and 7.2 every day of those four tests. Am I right?

If I am wrong and your pH is consistently between 6.8 and 7.2, then you are on track to restoring your health. Keep doing exactly what you are doing. You will get well!

I had a person that I met tell me that she was seeing a doctor in the USA who had 100% success rate in reversing cancer. When I asked what he was telling her to do, it was exactly what I am describing here.

If your pH is not in the ideal zone, then what can you do? Remember that minerals are key to the pH equation. From now on, you will want to make your food and drink choices be ones that are high in minerals, and low in sugar, or other acidic ingredients.

So, what foods do you believe have lots of minerals in them? If you guessed fresh, raw fruits and vegetables, you are right. The deeper the color, the more abundant the minerals.

Grasses like Wheatgrass and Barley grass are also rich in minerals, and especially sprouts of all kinds. I will be expanding on this in greater detail in a further chapter, but for now; the closer you can eat the way food is grown, the faster you will get well.

When I first heard about pH balancing, being inquisitive, I wanted to learn everything that I could about it. I took online courses. I bought books on the topic. I searched out where people were getting their knowledge from, and when food lists became conflicting, I searched it out even deeper. My husband teased me that I was getting my 'Ph.D.' in pH balancing.

I want you to know that you don't need your 'Ph.D' in pH balancing, in order to get well. Just choose fresh raw vegetables as the main food that you consume. One tip to keep in mind, is that mushrooms are not a vegetable, they are a fungus... not a good choice.

Before we go on to the 2nd half of the 'pH.D', it is important to understand that the 'D' part is the critical other half of the equation. They go hand in hand with each other. You will not be able to consistently maintain your pH in the healthy range, without addressing this next section. Many have tried and all have failed.

Taking Out the Garbage

The 'D' part of the 'pH.D'. acronym, represents one of the most important components in getting well from cancer. You need to Detoxify, or as I like to say "Get the Garbage out".

Here are a few facts:

- It is impossible to become pH balanced while you have a heavy toxic load in your body.
- Toxins are the breeding ground for disease, parasites and ill health.
- You will always have some level of toxins in your body. Every day, as your body breaks down the food that you eat, as well as when it replaces the old blood and cells, it creates debris. (toxins)

- Like laundry, the goal is to stay on top of the load, so that it doesn't pile up. Only with toxins, the ramifications are much more important.

There are two components to detoxification;

1. Stop adding as many toxins as possible, into your body.

2. Remove the toxins that you currently have, as well as the ones that develop from everyday life.

So, let's start first by avoiding as much as possible, adding more toxins into your already sick body.

How might you be unknowingly doing this?

Our skin being the largest organ of the body, will absorb whatever you rub or spray onto it. It will go directly into your bloodstream.

What are you putting onto your skin?

Here is a list of items that often have toxic ingredients; deodorant, talcum powder, perfume, moisturizing cream, toothpaste, shampoo, hair dye, styling gel, chlorine from your shower or bath, air fresheners, chemicals from dry cleaning clothes, mosquito spray, suntan lotion, cleaning supplies, soap for body, hands, clothes, dishes, as well as antibacterial wipes or gels when you enter stores and hospitals.

Natural alternatives can be found for most of the previous items.

My personal rule is; if I wouldn't want to eat it after looking at the ingredients, then I wouldn't want to ingest it through my skin, especially if it is put under the arms (lymph nodes), or on the hands or feet.

Whatever you rub onto the bottom of your feet, goes immediately into your body system. One way you can experience this principal is by rubbing a piece of garlic onto the bottom of the feet and see how long until you taste it in your mouth.

Next question is; what are you ingesting? Packaged foods are notorious for health destroying chemicals, especially things like aspartame and your worst enemy MSG.

If you eat only raw, organic fruits and vegetables in their natural, freshly picked condition, and no packaged food at all, you are welcome to skip over the next couple of pages, or you are welcome to read them, in order to remind you of why this is your pattern.

Yes, fresh, organic fruits and vegetables is what someone who either has cancer, or who is seeking to lower their chances of developing it, should be eating, but I am not naïve. I know that you get invited over to a friend's home, or you go out to restaurants, or you just get a 'hankering' for something unhealthy; so, I am providing you with this information as you transition to the healthiest way to live.

If I had my way, MSG would be outlawed, but I don't. So, I will warn you what other names it goes by. Next you will find the well-hidden, list of many different names for MSG.

Hidden Sources of MSG

The glutamate manufacturers and the processed food industries are always on a quest to disguise MSG that has been added to food items. Below is a partial list of the most common names for disguised MSG.

Additives that always contain MSG

Monosodium Glutamate
Hydrolyzed Vegetable Protein
Hydrolyzed Protein
Hydrolyzed Plant Protein
Plant Protein Extract
Sodium Caseinate
Calcium Caseinate
Yeast Extract
Textured Protein
Autolyzed Yeast
Hydrolyzed Oat Flour

Additives that frequently contain MSG

Malt Extract
Malt Flavoring
Bouillon
Broth
Stock
Flavoring

Natural Flavoring
Natural Beef or Chicken Flavoring
Seasoning
Spices

Additives that may contain MSG or other excito-toxins

Carrageenan
Enzymes
Soy Protein Concentrate
Soy Protein Isolate
Whey Protein Concentrate

As I endeavored to avoid MSG, I was amazed at all of the places that it is in. Often people think that it is found only in Chinese food. Yes, a lot of Chinese Restaurants use MSG to enhance the flavor, but most other restaurants and especially fast food outlets, also do.

Why?

Two reasons; it is a flavor enhancer as well as very addictive, so you will crave the food and hot drinks from that particular restaurant. Yes, it is even sometimes added to coffee and hot chocolate.

Have you ever wondered why Campbell's soup is "Mmm Good"? It is loaded with MSG.

Aspartame is worse for you than sugar... and sugar feeds cancer. If you would prefer to develop Alzheimer's along with having cancer, then this will aide in that quest.

If you are looking for a natural sweetener as you transition through your taste buds adjusting to the pleasures of fresh, raw fruits and vegetable, then use Stevia. Just be aware that some boxes of Stevia have added ingredients besides just plain Stevia. Yes, you may pay a bit more, but for your health, buy only pure Stevia.

Herbicides, Pesticides and GMO Foods are loaded with chemicals that dump a great deal of toxins into your system with each mouthful of food.

If you cannot locate organic or non-sprayed fresh fruits and vegetables, then it is important to wash them well either with a vegetable cleaner or else by mixing freshly squeezed lemon juice and 2 tablespoons of Celtic salt into your wash water. Let your produce sit in it for 15 – 20 minutes. Rinse well and then they can be used or stored in the fridge.

GMO foods are not only toxic, but they have the added part that the chromosomes have been altered, so they are not even the same produce.

Hair dyes and perms – There has been a direct correlation between black hair dye and lymphoma, I know that the hair dye chemicals as well as the perm chemicals, do get into your system via the skin. What is scary for me is that it goes in where our brain is. Yikes!!! Is curly hair really worth it, or is covering up the grey's that important to jeopardize your recovery? I say stick to your natural hair coloring, as you gracefully age.... especially if you already have cancer.

Vaccinations – Have you ever researched of what is put into vaccinations? If you haven't, then when you are well and have the extra time to spend on additional research, look into it. In the meantime, just trust me. You do not want this toxic soup injected into you.

That is the 'biggies' of where I would start to avoid adding more to your toxic load.

The 2nd part of detoxification is to help your body slowly release the toxins through following the information on the next few pages. It is extremely important to not skip over this part.

When my tumor marker was not getting worse, but it also was not improving, I was happy that it was not getting worse, but I also knew that there was something more that I needed to do in order to reverse the cancer.

My husband and I knew that I needed to help my body by removing the toxins in a major way, so we started to research our options.

We chose to go to a health retreat that specialized in detoxification. It cost a lot of money, but back in 2007, we didn't know some of the things that I will be sharing in the following pages.

If you choose to go somewhere to detoxify, make sure that juice fasting is a part of the program. Some health retreat places are just a healthy version of a spa, and do not focus on detoxification at the deep level that you need.

You will still want to read the different ways to detoxify, as over the years, you will want to stay on top of keeping your blood and organs clean. Also make sure to read about activated charcoal before you go to one, as I highly encourage you to take some with you.

Some Ways to Detoxify

Ok, let's look at what things you can do to assist your body in removing the toxins so you can move towards getting well.

What do you think of when you hear the word detox? A lot of people think of cleaning out the colon. Yes, our colon being cleaned out of years of debris is very important, but you also want to address a lot more than just your colon.

What is the largest organ that we have? Let's start there.

Our skin - Dry skin brushing is one of the best ways to remove dead, dry skin and to increase the circulation. When you remove the dead skin that is clogging your pores, you allow the skin to expel toxins.

Another way to help your body to detoxify through your skin is to do a daily hot and then cold shower. You do hot for three minutes and follow by cold for thirty seconds. Repeat three times in a row each day.

Another great way to assist your skin in flushing out the toxins, is by using a sauna/steam bath and then follow with a cold shower.

Before I go into how to detoxify the other organs, I think it is wise to introduce you to my friend 'Activated Charcoal'.

Activated Charcoal – If I could have only one item in my first aid kit, it would be activated charcoal. We carry it in our 5th wheel, my knapsack, the car and anytime I travel with a suitcase, it goes in. I have even found it helps me with restless leg syndrome, because allergies and/or toxins play a big part in this aggravating syndrome.

Anyone who has cancer or any other major illness, will find it helpful to have on hand, as it absorbs toxins in the body. In fact, if in the future you request to work with me either one on one, or through our online program, I will request you get some to have on hand.

When my husband Raven, and I went to the detox retreat, I was so grateful that I had packed it, because as I started to do some deep cleansing, toxins that I had put into my body almost thirty years previously, started to get pulled out from my body fat, and into my bloodstream. Taking the activated charcoal really helped me through those challenging times.

I was happy I had it on hand when a friend who is deathly allergic to nuts ate some Pesto pizza before he realized that it was made from pine nuts. I had him drink the activated charcoal mixed into water and 15 minutes later, he drank another glass. He had no reaction at all.

I am extremely allergic to bee stings, but because I had not been stung in years, I stopped keeping my antihistamines up to date. One day when I was alone, I was stung by a bee. My arm began to swell, and became red and itchy around the sting. I immediately drank some activated charcoal, as well as I mixed-up some with a little water to make a paste and covered the sting area with it. It stopped the swelling, as well as the redness from spreading. The itching started to subside. The next day, you could not even tell that I had been stung.

If you would like more information about Activated Charcoal, be sure to go to **www.AreYouinBalance.com** where you can receive a free download of a mini e-book that I wrote especially for you, covering:

How to use it
How much to use
How often to use
Cautions
Where to purchase it

I have on purpose kept the booklet focused on only the information that I feel you need right now, so as to not overwhelm you. Later on, when you are back in health, and not feeling overwhelmed, there are some great books out there that you can get from a health food store that describe all of the many uses for it.

Ok, now I feel comfortable on telling you ways to draw the toxins out.

Blood – Life is in the blood.

Fresh raw beet juice will cleanse the blood. A caution about beet juice; only juice a couple of ounces of beets at a time as it is a strong cleanser and may detoxify you too quickly. That could be dangerous to flood yourself with more toxins than your body can handle. It is best mixed with other vegetables like carrots. I have included some great recipes in two more chapters.

The herb Red Clover is a great, safe blood cleanser. I buy it in a capsule and then empty the herbs from two capsules, into hot water for a tea and do it three times each day. If you happen to be using a blood thinner called Warfarin, Red Clover is not recommended until you check with your health practitioner first.

Astragalus is also wonderful for people with cancer, as it not only cleanses the blood, but it helps to protect the immune system and improves digestion. I often see digestive issues in people with cancer.

Another way to cleanse the blood, is to make some raw, unsweetened almond milk. Next, juice some organic dark grapes. Then, combine one cup of each into a two-cup mug. It doesn't look very appetizing, but after stirring it, it is very tasty, especially if you have both ingredients chilled first.

Colon – Keeping the colon clean is critical for helping to not re-absorb toxins that you have loosened up. It is also important to keep clean in order to help your body to absorb the much-needed nutrients that are essential to getting well. Following are a few ways to cleanse your colon.

Saline Cleanse – First thing in the morning before you have had anything to eat or drink, except plain water, mix together 4 cups of hot water and 2 tsp of unrefined sea salt. (My favorite brand is called 'Real Salt' by Redmond's) Let it sit until it cools down to the place that you can drink all four cups of water within 10 minutes.

If you know that there is not any hope of you being able to currently drink four cups of warm water within ten minutes, or if this is for a child or a very petite person, then you can half the recipe. Use two cups of water and one teaspoon of salt. Keep in mind that if you are an adult and choose to start with half of the recipe, in order to get the best cleanse, you will want to increase it to the full amount as soon as you are able to.

Drink it down (tastes like chicken noodle soup... if you have a good imagination) and stay close to a washroom. The salt acts like a magnet as it travels through your body, pulling toxins from the lymph and your colon. You will have gushes of watery feces be expelled.

Wait to make sure that you have expelled all that you are going to, before the next step.

Next, it is important to replace the electrolytes that you have just lost. One of the most pleasant ways of doing this, is by juicing 1 lemon, 2 oranges and 1 – 2 grapefruits to make a two-cup juice. It is so delicious and refreshing.

This Saline Cleanse can be repeated each morning for a week, but I would not do it longer than two weeks in a row.

Coffee Enema – An enema can be done in the privacy of your own home, as often as needed throughout the day. Dr. Max Gerson advocated a coffee enema every four hours in the beginning, and then increasing it as the body starts to dissolve the cancerous tissue over the next three or four months. Dr. Gerson discovered that the coffee enema helps to encourage the liver to flush the toxins out by opening up the bile ducts of the gallbladder. It is very important to use organic coffee for this.

Enemas also help to relieve pain because pain is caused from toxins.

Can you have an enema without adding the coffee? Absolutely. It just won't stimulate the bile ducts to open as much, but it will help to keep the colon clean as you release toxins, or if you become constipated.

Dr. Lorraine Day describes in her video's, how she did enemas without the coffee on her journey with cancer, as she didn't feel comfortable adding the coffee. Personally, I am hyper sensitive to caffeine, so I also would forgo the coffee.

Colonic – A colonic is a high enema done by a professional Hydro Therapist. In the first couple of years after I was diagnosed with Lymphoma, I used this as part of my healing regime. I would have continued longer, but the cost was hard for me to keep doing.

Some offer to add either chlorophyll or wheatgrass to the water that you hold in your colon before you expel it. Personally, I would do a couple with plain water first, so that you practice holding it before spending the extra on adding the chlorophyll or wheatgrass.

I highly recommend that you find a professional to do this treatment for you, as there are people who have no training who offer it.

Gallbladder Flush – Start off by fasting on freshly made raw apple juice or grapefruit juice. Fast for 24 – 48 hours on this juice. For those with low blood sugar issues or if you have a yeast infection, then use the grapefruit juice instead of the apple, as it has less natural occurring sugar.

If you need to use the grapefruit juice instead of the apple, you will need to supplement with some malic acid and magnesium which the apple juice has naturally occurring.

Just before going to bed, as you are getting ready to stop the fast, mix together ½ cup olive oil with ½ cup freshly made lemon or grapefruit juice. Drink this and then lie down on your right side for half an hour before hopping into bed for the night.

In the morning you should have a bowel movement. If not, do an enema. This can be repeated a 2nd night, making sure to fast on nothing but apple or grapefruit juice all through the day again.

Kidney – Dandelion leaves are great for cleansing the kidneys. Add some to your juice each day. A wonderful Chinese herbal formula that I used when I developed a kidney infection is called KBC. My doctor wanted me to use antibiotics, but because 'anti' means against and 'biotic' means life, I wanted to go with health building herbs instead. It really helped address the root cause, rather than just the symptom.

Liver – First thing each morning (except the days you are planning on doing a saline cleanse), before you have anything to eat or drink (except for plain water); freshly squeeze half of a lemon into 2 cups warm water. This is an excellent drink rather than coffee, and can be safely done every day.

This is so good for your liver as lemon is a natural cleanser and a practice to do for the rest of your life.

Activated Charcoal will absorb toxins in the liver extremely well. In fact, if by accident a person eats a deadly poisonous mushroom called Death Cap, they have found that only two things can save the person's life; Milk Thistle because it protects the liver from the poison and Activated Charcoal because it absorbs the poison so that it doesn't destroy the liver.

Lungs – If you smoke, now is a good time to stop. There is no need to ask your body to work even harder than it needs to in order to get well.

Deep breathing when you are outside is a great way to help your body get more oxygen.

Spend time out in nature as much as you can, especially around evergreen trees like Pine, Fir, Cypress, Spruce, Cedar.

If it is at all possible, the best place to live is away from the larger cities, preferably in the country. That has been our priority and God has continually provided a place for us to live a country lifestyle.

Steam baths are another great way to help your lungs detoxify, as it helps to break up the mucus in the lungs. But be cautious of not staying longer than 15 minutes at a time in it. Always follow it with a brief cold shower,

Lymphatic – Rebounding is one of the very best ways to cleanse your lymphatic system as it is one of the few ways to open and close the lymphatic system. Start off bouncing for a minute or two. Gradually increase until you can comfortably bounce for 15 – 20 minutes at a time, or else you can bounce for 5 minutes three times a day.

Another great way to help the lymph system cleanse is by having a massage therapist who is trained in lymphatic drainage to do your massage.

I have personally found that applying Frankincense Therapeutic Essential Oil to the skin where my lymph nodes are, on one day, then the next day applying a mixture of Frankincense, Myrrh and Sage, really worked quickly to decrease the swelling in my lymph nodes. You mix 10 drops of Frankincense, 5 drops of Myrrh and 3 drops of Sage with a bit of mixing oil, before applying to your skin.

I found that using a shot glass to mix these together helped a lot. I would dip my fingers into the mixture and apply it until all of it was used-up. Continue to alternate between using just Frankincense, and applying the mixture.

Recently, I discovered that one of my favorite cancer herbal combinations is also useful to detoxify the Lymphatic System. You get a double blessing from a product called E-Tea, which I describe more in Section 6.

Warning: If you have a brain tumor, it is not advisable to use this, until after the tumor has shrunk.

So now you have some ideas on how you can cleanse your skin, blood, colon, gallbladder, kidneys, liver, lungs and lymphatic system, either as your first detox, or else as a subsequent detox.

My husband and I, chose to go to a detox retreat. Yes it cost us a lot to attend, but not only did we gain a lot of value from the daily health lectures and videos, but I was also grateful that I was able to experience all of the detox methods that we did while we were there, as they made a huge difference in my healing.

If finances are not an issue, personally, I would recommend that you go to somewhere like the Gerson Clinic in Mexico, or Hippocrates Health Institute in Florida.

But if you do not have the money to go to a detox retreat/clinic, you can do what I learned about when we got home and now do a few times a year.

Within a few weeks of coming home from the detox retreat, I was introduced to a product called Bod-E-Klenz. As a natural health consultant, I was extremely impressed by what it contained. It had everything to cleanse all areas of the body (except the skin). It also had herbs which helped to rebuild the body and the pH levels.

Since 2007, I have used it not only for my clients, but many, many times on myself as I like to do a cleanse 3 - 4 times a year, which I cannot afford the cost of going to a detox retreat each time.

Recently, our Canadian government decided to no longer allow us to purchase Bod-E Klenz as a kit. Thankfully, we can still do one of two things; it can be purchased for personal use from the USA, or the herbs that made up the kit, can (as of this writing) be purchased individually, with a tiny bit of modification. In the USA, it is called Dieter's Cleanse. You can safely take it up to four months in a row, if you feel the need to. Don't worry, you still eat your regular meals, with the knowledge that the closer you stick to the foods described under nutrition, the faster you will get well.

I would be happy to help you get this excellent kit or individual components at my discount. Just go to **http://HelloHealth.mynsp.com**, to see what is available in your country.

Heavy Metals – Do you have any mercury fillings in your mouth? I know first-hand on how much this can deplete your immune system.

Back in 1987, before it was common knowledge that the amalgam fillings in our mouth, could leak mercury into our body, I started to develop severe allergies to so many foods, that I started to be afraid of eating.

I lost an incredible amount of weight. I also started to find myself losing strength to the place that as a waitress, I could not even carry a coffee pot to serve my customers.

The final warning that I was rapidly going downhill, was when I could no longer even open a car door. I felt like I was slowly dying.

My boyfriend at the time, was an avid reader, and stumbled upon the symptoms that mercury poisoning can cause. I was definitely displaying the symptoms.

As I had a mouth full of fillings from when I had cancer as a child, I knew that some of them were twenty-three years old, which put them at high risk of leaching into my blood stream.

I searched all over the city we lived in, to find a dentist who understood what I was talking about, when I requested to have the fillings changed over to porcelain. I was thrown out of a few dentist offices at even suggesting that my fillings were causing my symptoms.

I finally found a dentist who not only was aware of the health risk, but more importantly, he understood how to safely remove the fillings, without dumping even more poison into my already compromised body.

Within a month of removing them, as well as assisting my body on removing the mercury and other metals that were playing havoc on my immune system, my strength started to slowly return. It took a lot longer for my allergies to subside, and some still trouble me if I overdo it, but at least I knew without a shadow of doubt, what the culprit was.

While we are talking about dental health risks, it has been shown that root canals also possess threats to our immune system. In fact, there are some natural health cancer doctors, who will not work with you until you have removed both your amalgam fillings, as well as your root canals, due to the bacteria growth that can seep into your bloodstream from root canals.

It was discovered that when a person has two or more root canals, their chance of developing cancer, is higher than the general population. I personally had three.

Back to discussing heavy metals.

It is important to remove heavy metals from your body. One of the safest ways to help your body is by having a baking soda bath.

Here is how you do them; mix 1 ½ cups of baking soda into a hot bath. When I say a hot bath, I am referring to keeping the temperature between 105 – 110 degrees Fahrenheit during a 30-minute soak.

Make sure to keep the trunk of your body in the water during the bath.

Scrub your body during the bath with a loofa sponge, always stroking towards the heart.

Keep a cool cloth or ice next to the tub to be used to keep your head cool.

Shower after the soak to rinse your skin off.

This is best done when there is someone to monitor how you are doing to make sure that you haven't passed out.

The water will turn grey as the toxins come out. out. Do this every second or third night, until the water stays clear.

Another way to remove heavy metals is by using a heavy metals detox in the form of herbs. Cilantro is one of the main ingredients of the one that I recommend.

Always work on removing heavy metals AFTER most of the other toxins have been removed first, or else your body may have a challenge on handling the extra load of dumping heavy metals into it as well.

Early in my career, I had a client who really wanted to do a heavy metal cleanse. We started it before she had done any other body cleanses. She felt awful after a couple of days of doing it.

I stopped her from continuing. We did a Bod-E-Klenz and she felt wonderful. So good in fact, that she wanted to repeat it. After checking with the company, I was assured that she could repeat it up to four months in a row. She ended up doing it for three months and felt better and better. Afterwards, she went back to the heavy metal cleanser, and breezed through it this time.

In the meantime, you can add some cilantro and kelp to your diet as they are great absorbers of heavy metals.

It is also important to be using healthy oils on a daily basis, even when you are not attempting to rid your body of heavy metals. Not only does it bind the heavy metals together for removal of them, but is also great for rebuilding the immune system.

My #1 preference is flax seeds or flax seed oil, as they are high in Omega 3, which is good for fighting cancer. It is important to not use flax seed oil for cooking though. Instead use coconut or extra virgin olive oil, to cook with.

Parasites – Parasites are not just in third world countries. Yes, you can pick up parasites from travelling, but our pets also are a prevalent source of parasites, especially if they are allowed on the furniture, or the bed.

Another source of parasites is eating pork, fish, eating in restaurants, working in the garden without gloves on, walking barefoot where birds have been (the beach or grass).

Most people have parasites and do not even know it. Having cancer, it is important to remove them, as you do not want to share your nutrients with these critters.

There are lots of parasite cleanses available. You are welcome to go to **http://HelloHealth.mynsp.com,** for the one that I like to use, or else you can use any other ones that you trust the manufacturer. I stumbled upon a great one while living in Mexico.

Depending on how many days the kit is; you need to time the start of taking it before the full moon of that month. If it is a ten day one, then start five days before the full moon. If it is a fifteen day one, then start it seven days before the full moon.

The reason it is often recommended that you start it before a full moon and carry on through to an equal amount after the full moon, is because it is thought that parasites are more active during this time frame.

Repeat the kit the following month so as to destroy any new parasites that have hatched, also keeping in mind when the full moon is.

It is a good idea to have everyone in your family do a parasite cleanse at the same time, and especially if you share a bed with your spouse, as you do not want to re-infect yourself.

Parasite cleanses should be done at least twice a year after each detox, when you know that the elimination channels are open.

Emotional and Spiritual Cleanse – Most people do not think of their emotions and their spiritual wellness, as needing to be cleansed. But it is very important to address these two areas in order to recover fully.

I once knew a woman who had appeared to be cancer free for ten years at that point. She was the only person that I personally knew who had gone the medical route, and lived for ten years.

When her cancer returned, she asked me to work with her. I knew that she was a very confrontational person, as well as having an incredible amount of anger and bitterness in her, which I knew would prevent her from healing. She also confided in me that she felt like her husband was just waiting for her to die.

I felt sad knowing that she had major work ahead of her in order to heal. I was not convinced that she would follow what I recommended, let alone work on her emotional issues, so I decided to ask her questions to tell me how willing she was to be healed.

I knew that her cancer had 'returned', because she had done chemotherapy, and had never worked on her emotional issues, nor her spiritual ones.

Unfortunately, I could tell by her answers, that she was not willing to do all that it would take to turn her health around.

She was convinced that her husband was to blame for her cancer, and that he needed to change, not her.

She had so much unforgiveness, and anger in her heart, that I knew even if she would follow the physical health restoring principals, her refusal to address her emotions, would prevent her from turning her health around.

Sure enough, her health kept on deteriorating until unfortunately she passed away.

So, what can you do to have emotional cleansing?

You will notice that the last four letters of the acronym, all has to do with the emotions. Make sure to not skip over them.

Find a good Christian counsellor who will walk you through letting go of anger, bitterness and unforgiveness.

I have a written exercise that I have my clients do, which helps them with any unforgiveness, that they may still be holding onto. (I am a Christian counsellor) You are welcome to obtain a copy of this exercise by going to my website **www.AreYouinBalance.com**

With regards to spiritual cleansing; are you angry with God?

Has this cancer journey brought you into a closer relationship with Him or has it been one of distance?

Do you trust Him?

I love a song by Babbie Mason, called 'Trust His Heart'. You can look it up on Youtube, but here are the words that I most resonated with.

"God is too wise to be mistaken
God is too good to be unkind
So, when you can't understand,
When you can't see His plan,
When you can't trace His hand,
Trust His heart."

Two weeks before I was diagnosed with cancer, God woke me up at 4 am and gave me a book to write called; 'Where Was God When I Needed Him Most?'

During this morning chat, He walked me through scenario after scenario of different times that He had been there for me in my time of need. He was preparing me to receive the news of having cancer. I knew that if He could be trusted through all of those other times, then I could trust Him to walk with me on this journey as well.

What about you? When has God been there for you previously? How has He proven that He is trustworthy? Ask Him to show you.

Under the letter "A", of section 5, you will get some additional ideas that will help you to be reminded of His goodness.

Lastly, you may want to watch testimonials of others who have had incredible experiences of seeing God working in their lives, or read their books. One of my favorite books is by David Gates, called; 'Mission Pilot'. Of course, you can read one of my books as well; either 'Where Was God When I Needed Him Most?', or 'So Lord, Where to Next?' (once they are available)

Section 4
Rolling Up
Your Sleeves

Breath of Life

Let's start with the first letter of the acronym A.N.S.W.E.R.S. The 'A' stands for Air.

We can only last an average of three minutes without air, before we would die. We become lightheaded and may faint when our brain is deprived of oxygen for even a short period of time. We receive permanent brain damage after just four minutes without oxygen.

Besides not developing brain damage, light headedness, or dying, why else do we need air?

We rely on air to supply the body's need for oxygen, and to eliminate carbon dioxide from the body.

Carbon dioxide can kill us humans. Plants love it, but it is detrimental to us. They give off oxygen that we need, in exchange for the carbon dioxide, which they thrive on.

A pretty fair exchange, don't you think? It gets me thinking about the wisdom of living in a garden, back at the beginning of time.

One potted plant per one hundred square feet of living space, will help to keep the air inside your home or office the healthiest. The best plants for this are; Aloe Vera, Corx, Ivy, Philodendrons, Snake Plants, Spider Plants and Peace Lilies.

Air is either negatively charged or positively charged.

Unlike what you may initially think, it is better to have a high amount of negatively charged ions in the air that you breathe compared to positively charged ions.

Negative ions do a few things; it helps to rebuild the immune system, it lifts depression and heals the body, whereas positive ions will give you headaches and make you feel tired and irritable.

Outside air has a negative charge, with country air normally having double the negative ions than city air. Normally inside air has a lot more positive ions, than outside.

Only pure, negatively charged air, can make pure blood. Pure blood is where healing occurs. What are some ways to take in more negatively charged air from outside?

- Go outside daily for a walk in clean fresh air for 30 – 45 minutes.

- As often as possible walk out in nature and especially around the evergreen trees; (fir, pine, cedar, balsam), as they give off life-giving properties, which build health.

- Spend time in parks. Lie in the grass (I did a lot of that as a child, and still love to.)

- Go for a walk in the mountains. Even just sitting in a garden, taking in the aroma's, will give you benefits.

- If you can, go camping in a tent. Tents allow you to inhale close to the maximum amount of negatively charged ions while you sleep, especially if you have pitched your tent in the forest.

  Placing your tent directly on grass or the ground is much better than on a cement slab.

  As a child, my parents took me camping a lot. We slept in a tent in the middle of campgrounds with an abundance of tall pine trees. Pine trees are the richest evergreen tree of negative ions. Still to this day, I feel my very best camping in the forest. I sleep way better than any other place.

- For those of you who just cannot fathom sleeping in a tent, and resorts are more your thing, treat yourself to one of those cabana's perched over the ocean. Pounding waves, are abundant in negative ions, as well.

Years ago, while in Saint Lucia, I was able to experience sleeping over the ocean in a cabana, and had an awesome sleep.

- Sitting at the beach, or by a river, even in winter months, and taking in deep breaths of the ocean air will work on improving your immune system.

  Through my teen years, I loved to escape down to the ocean whenever I felt like I needed time alone. Sometimes, I would spend hours just taking in the beauty.

Now that I know about the healing properties of the forest and the beach, I understand that even though I did not know it at the time, these were some ways that my body was healing me as a child from cancer.

Forests, the beach and especially waterfalls, are high in negatively charged air, so even if you are not able to find anyone to go for a walk, or go camping with you out in the forests, and you don't want to go alone, then head to the beach, kick off your shoes and walk barefoot along the sand.

In the spring and summer, I kick off my shoes and walk barefoot on the grass as often as I can. Just watch out for prickles, and in our area, I also need to watch for cacti.

The best place to live is out in the country. If moving to the country is not possible, then spend as much time out in nature as possible, even if it means living in a trailer in nature, then do it. Just make sure to keep the windows and doors open as much as possible. This is especially important while you are healing.

It is important to replace the positive ions in the house with fresh negative ions, especially while you are sleeping.

What are some ways to replace the positive ions in your home?

Raven and I, all year long, keep our bedroom window open, even if only a few inches in the winter months.

Before going to bed at night, turn off any heat you may have on. Then either open your bedroom window or else you can open another window, as long as you keep your bedroom door open, to allow the poor-quality air to be moved out.

Do this all year long, even if it is just a few inches. This will remove the stale, positively charged air and let in the fresh, negative ions from outside.

You will find that your sleep will improve greatly.

In spring, summer, and fall, keep your doors and windows open as long as possible each day. In winter, before we start up any heat in the morning, we open up the doors and windows for about fifteen to thirty minutes to allow a good exchange of air to happen.

Cigarette smoke, besides being toxic to breathe, removes negative ions, so allowing someone to smoke in your home or car, is detrimental to your health building journey, as it will deplete your immune system.

It is important to take in some deep breaths of quality air through out each and every day.

This is how you do proper deep breathing:

Lie down flat, or sit in a comfortable position.

Put one hand on your belly just below your ribs and the other hand on your chest.

Take a deep breath in through your nose, and let your belly push your hand out.

Breathe out through pursed lips as if you were whistling.

Repeat this type of deep breathing for a minimum of three times.

Rebuilding Your Immune System

The second letter in this acronym is 'N', which stands for Nutrition.

I have been asked if the Keto Diet, is the best one for healing from cancer?

There are a lot of people, including doctors who are saying that the very best diet to be on for helping your body to destroy cancer, is the Keto Diet. So, let's look at it together to see if this is what you should follow.

What is the Keto Diet? It is a diet that recognizes that sugar is not good for us. It also recognizes that refined flour is also not good for us. It is a diet that attempts to force your body to burn the stored fat rather than the preferred carbohydrates, that it would normally choose to burn.

It forces the body into what is called 'Ketosis'. As I do not want to overload you with information that will not truly help with your decision if this is the best diet to follow, I will not go into it. You can always look it up online if you will not be able to rest until you know more than I provide here.

So, let's take apart the foods that you are encouraged to not eat as well as what they say to eat on a Keto Diet.

Eliminate sugar. This is definitely what a person who has been diagnosed with cancer or any other disease needs to do. Sugar lowers the immune system, as well as it 'lights up' cancer cells, and encourages them to grow.

Eliminate refined flour. Refined flour can cause inflammation in the body, which is one of the contributing factors for developing cancer.

I also personally discourage bread, unless you have freshly grown your own grains and milled it yourself. The reason that I say to only eat grains that you have freshly grown, is because stored grains often have developed mold on them while in storage, which of course you do not need more toxins that need to be removed.

The diet cuts carbohydrates way back, and encourages the person to eat more protein and fats. So, what are carb's?

There are two types of carb's; simple and complex. Simple carbs are foods that breakdown quickly in your body, like sugar, bread, and most fruit. Complex carb's break down slower due to the high fiber content.

The Keto diet advocates eating more fat and protein. Fat and protein in itself are not bad for us.

Depending on the source of fat and protein, would be the deciding factor. If it is from animal protein and fat, that is not healthy with or without cancer.

If the fat is from things like flax seeds/oil, avocados, coconut butter, olives, then that is healthy.

If the protein is from things like spinach, beans, lentils, then this is also healthy for you. The only exception to this, is if you are currently having digestive issues, you may want to hold off on the beans, as they are harder to digest. If you find that lentils also bother you, then wait on them as well.

When you go to re-introduce them, start with the lentils first, and add beans back into your diet last.

An excellent source of protein that is easily digested is barley juice, as well as chlorella. Both of these are rich in alkalizing chlorophyll, and come in a powder form. Of course, organic and without fillers is what you want to look for. I use to use and recommend Enerex Just Barley, but unfortunately, they have stopped producing it. AIM is a reputable company. Let me know if you find another great one.

I have recently bought Seven Hills Chlorella on Amazon, and find it a great brand. I plan on putting some links for products that I recommend on our website; **www.AreYouinBalance.com**

What about fruit and complex carbs?

Fresh raw fruit has a lot of health building enzymes. Eating them raw is healthy.

Complex carbs are your vegetables, brown rice, oats, beans and lentils. Are they healthy? Absolutely!

The more you eat your vegetables raw, the better, as cooked foods are dead food. When you heat your food over 117 degrees, you destroy the enzymes in them.

We need enzymes in order for the body to be able to utilize minerals, and we need minerals for our body to be able to use vitamins.

Digestive issues can happen when we do not have the necessary enzymes to break down the food. I have noticed that people who have developed cancer, often have digestive issues. So be gentle on your body, by eating as much raw as possible.

Lastly, studies have shown that when a person is in remission from cancer, if they eat more than 25% of their food cooked, the cancer returned.

Here are some important tips;

- While getting well from cancer, the very best diet to follow is fresh raw fruit and vegetables, flax seed oil, and 13 cups of freshly prepared juices spread throughout the day.

I noticed that going 100% raw, was when my cancer reversed the fastest. I also know that when Veronica was given two weeks to live, she also went 100% raw. My conclusion is that the closer you stick to 100% raw, the more your body has the tools to heal you.

- It is important, once you are well, to still drink at least 4 cups of freshly made juice each day, which will also help you keep the 75 – 80% of your diet raw.

- Once you are well, or as you are working up to 100% raw, then this is what I found helpful; if you would like something warm to 'ADD' to your raw vegetables, add in some Basmati brown rice, a baked yam or a baked potato (these three can be pleasantly topped with flax seed oil, freshly squeezed lemon juice, raw green onions, fresh garlic, raw broccoli, sundried tomatoes, or any other raw vegetables you happen to have in your fridge).

- If you want to add something warm to your fresh raw fruit, cook up some slow cooked oats, and enjoy it with plain rice milk, or almond milk, a chopped apple and some cinnamon.

- Any foods you want to cook or heat up, always use the stove, a slow cooker or a toaster oven.

Never use a microwave, as it is one of the unhealthiest ways to heat up any food or liquid. Microwaving foods not only has the nutrients greatly diminished, but it is also toxic to the body, due to the molecule structure of the food being changed while it is being cooked. Don't even warm up a cup of water with a microwave. There is a very important reason why Russia banned microwaves from their country!!!

- Once you are well, then you can slowly add in some fresh raw nuts and seeds, as well as some lentils and occasionally some beans. (black beans, pinto beans, lima beans, garbanzo beans, aka chick peas)

- What about dairy? A lot of diets recommend dairy and especially cheese as a healthy source of protein.

  Dairy is not only full of antibiotics, and hormones, but it is also health destroying due to the extremely low pH to it, with cheese being one of the worst.

  A study was done independently by both Dr. T. Colin Campbell, as well as Dr. Caldwell Esselstyn. They both discovered that they were able to turn cancer on and off with cheese alone. Pretty scary!!!

- Protect your meal time from being one of stress. Don't rush through a meal. Instead take your time and thoroughly enjoy every mouthful of food.

> Studies have shown that even if we eat a perfectly nutritious meal, but are stressed at the time of eating it, we lose two-thirds of the nutrients from entering our body.

REMEMBER! You are eating foods to save your life NOT for entertainment.

The Power of Juicing

The goal of the foods that you will be consuming, is to flood your body with nutrients that heal and rebuild as God created it to do.

Juicing is the fastest way to do this, which also helps your digestive system, have a break. Due to most people who have cancer also having problems with their digestive system, it is almost impossible to eat enough food to get the level of nutrients needed to assist your body to heal without the aid of juicing.

Raw food is alive. It has the most amount of healing properties. Juicing is one of the easiest ways to consume more raw vegetables, while not feeling like a rabbit.

Often, I am asked if a person should only drink juice and no food, or do they eat meals as well.

You can do either. The most important thing is that you give your body the tools that it needs to heal, so don't skimp on the juices because you are too full from your meals. Your meals are to supplement the juices, rather than the juices supplementing your meals.

Joe Cross from 'Fat, Sick and Nearly Dead', consumed only freshly made juices for 60 days in an attempt to reverse an autoimmune disease that doctors could not help him with. Not only did he reverse this disease that no-one else had an answer for him, he also got off all of his medications. As an extra bonus, he lost 100 unwanted pounds. His DVD is listed as ones that I highly recommend.

If you are underweight or not willing to only juice, then I would encourage you to start having your juices as soon as you get up in the morning, and in between your meals.

For good digestion, do not drink anything including your juices with your meals. Instead wait two hours after your meal and no closer than half an hour before the next one.

Some people find sticking 100% to the juices is the easiest for them. Then I say go for it, but if you are on medications of any sort, work with a doctor to lower your prescriptions as your body repairs itself. This can happen very quickly.

Thirty to sixty days is the ideal amount of time to do only the juices without eating meals. But even thirty days will give your body an incredible healing kick-start.

Any juice fasts over three days, you will want to work either with a Naturopath or a Natural Health Consultant who is trained on the way to reintroduce food back into your stomach after a fast. This is VERY important.

As I want to keep this book as uncomplicated as possible, I will not go into the re-entering of food after a juice fast.

Instead, in our online course, I will go into how to do this in great detail, where I can answer questions along the way.

Why not start your day with the following juice; 1 lemon, 2 oranges and 1 – 2 grapefruits. This is done easiest with a citrus juicer. (as well as the least clean up)

For the rest of the day, choose vegetables and/or greens like spinach, kale, swiss chard, lettuce as the main ingredient.

To get started, here are a few recipes that I personally do;

One granny smith apple juiced with enough carrots juiced to make two cups of juice

6 oz. of spinach juice with 10 oz. of carrot juice

One of my favorites is; 1 lemon, 2 granny smith apples, ½ of a pineapple, 1 long English cucumber and enough spinach to make 4 cups of juice in total.

Another one that I really enjoy is; ½ of a small red cabbage, 1 green pepper, 4 red chard leaves, 4 handfuls of romaine lettuce, 4 granny smith apples and 4 handfuls of endive lettuce or any other nutrient rich lettuce (just not iceberg). This makes 4 cups of juice.

This one is Joe Cross's 'Mean Green' juice; 1 lemon, a couple tablespoons of fresh ginger, 2 long English cucumbers, 4 granny smith apples, 8 celery sticks and 12 – 16 kale leaves. This will make 4 – 5 cups of juice.

Another one to do, is 1 granny smith apple, 1 lemon, 3 small beets, and enough carrots to make 4 cups of juice... so good!

I think that I will go make that one right now.

Or try 2 granny smith apples, 1 cucumber, 6-8 sprigs mint, 6-8 leaves kale, 2 handfuls mixed greens, 1 lemon, peeled and juiced.

Huatulco, Mexico Verde Jugo (Green Juice); uses 500 ml freshly made orange juice, 2 guava's, 2 slices pineapple, 1 large handful of spinach, ½ stalk of celery and a small handful of parsley. Soooo refreshing in the heat.

Even though I would most likely get started with the above recipes, down the road when you are looking for new ones, Joe Cross has some great juice recipes, as well as healthy meal recipes on his website; ***www.rebootwithjoe.com***

Jugo Juice also has some awesome recipes. If you go to their website, you can write down what ingredients they use. They don't list how much of each, but as you follow the above recipes, you will get a feel for how much of each ingredient to use and of course you can adjust it to suit your taste.

The most important concept that you need to keep in mind is you are juicing for repair work, so make sure that you are keeping greens and vegetables as the main ingredients, rather than just fruits. This is especially important if you are currently a diabetic. You can lower the amounts of fruit, or eliminate them from your juice, and then eat them raw, between your juices, so as to retain the fiber and thus slow down the rate of the sugar entering your body.

You will be drinking thirteen juices a day during your healing process, and for at least six months after you are cancer free. After that, you will want to drink at least four cups of juice a day for the rest of your life.

Not only will you feel great and have more energy, but you are also actively keeping your body in the cancer free zone.

You may feel tempted to just stick to your favorite green juice along with the carrot and apple juice. I want to encourage you to rotate through the greens instead of sticking to just spinach or just kale. The reason for this is that each greens, have their own properties and you need to vary them at least once a week.

One way to rotate them, without giving up your favorite recipe is to use the same recipe, just change the greens that particular day. Swiss chard is a great switch for spinach, as they both are mild tasting.

If you would like my printable juice recipes pdf file, so that you can have it handy when you are making your juices, just go to my website **www.AreYouinBalance.com**, where you can download it.

I personally, have mine in a sheet protector, so that it is splatter friendly.

Following is some education of why you are using certain ingredients. I have included this for those days when you may not feel like drinking your juices. Hopefully, it will inspire you to drink up.

Carrot juice has been shown in studies to dissolve tumours.

Spinach is a power house of minerals and enzymes that have healing properties for the nervous system.

Carrot and spinach juice help replace the minerals that often are low when a person has cancer.

Granny smith apples have enzymes that work on cancer.

Cucumbers are very alkalizing.

Kale is the king of nutrients in green leafy vegetables.

Pineapple is great for upset stomachs as well as for digestive issues.

Beets help to rebuild the quality of your blood.

Lemons are alkalizing, as well as they help to cleanse the liver.

Lettuce, especially the dark green ones, are loaded with minerals that help to alkalize the body.

Personally, I make up 4 cups of one juice at a time and pour them into 2 cup jars, right to the top. Mason canning jars work well.

If you do not have enough juice to fill up both jars to the top, then split the juice between the two jars, and top them off with quality water. The other option is to juice some more of one of the ingredients to stretch it to the 4 cups. Cucumbers are a great one to juice extra of, as it is rich in liquids. Seal it and put them into the fridge. This way, I am only juicing 2 -3 times a day.

I love drinking each two cups with a straw. I got the idea to do that when watching Joe Cross's movie 'Fat, Sick and Nearly Dead'. Not 100% positive, but I believe that with a straw, the juice hits a different part of the taste buds that affects the enjoyment.

How much juice should you drink?

Dr. Lorraine Day, as well as The Gerson Clinic both say 13 cups per day; 1 citrus, 8 carrot and 4 greens. Joe Cross drank 10 cups of juice on his juice fast. (from his DVD) Personally when I first got started, I could not drink that much. Unfortunately, at that point in my research, I did not understand about pH balancing, so I drank my citrus and 4 cups of carrot with a granny smith apple. I never got to the green juices. This stopped my cancer from growing, but it did not reverse it.

From what I now know, I would have started with my citrus juice, then my greens and then my carrot juices, even if I only got 2 cups of carrot in as I built up to 8 cups of carrot.... Or even better yet, I would do 6 cups of greens and 6 cups of carrot. Carrots are important for breaking down the tumors, but the greens are critical for changing the alkaline environment.

I am often asked what type of juicer to buy.

When I first got started juicing, I went to Walmart and bought one for around $50. It had a stainless steel cutting disc as the base of a mesh filter basket. It is often called a centrifugal juicer.

It got me started but was a challenge for juicing leafy green vegetables. In fact, I couldn't do them.

I then had a friend who was selling her Juiceman Juicer, which STILL did not do the greens as it also was a centrifugal juicer, but at least the mouth to put the apple and carrots in, was larger.

Finally, after already spending close to $200 on these two juicers, I bought a Samson juicer, which has what is called an auger to crush the produce, rather than spinning them past a cutter. I was happy with the Samson choice. I got a lot more juice out of my produce, so it saved me money on my groceries. It even came with a 15-year warranty, so you know that it was quality.

The only parts that I was not crazy about, was two things;

1. I had to cut up my produce more, as the chute is pretty narrow, and

2. really juicy soft fruits like pineapple, watermelon and grapes, seemed to leak out, due to the design.

So, then I bought the one that I currently have, which is called a Hurom. It has all of the features of the Samson, except that it is upright, so the juicy, soft fruits, does not leak out the same way. It still has the issue of the narrow chute, but I finally found a solution for that.

When my husband's daughter was diagnosed with a brain tumor, we packed up our juicer and headed up to her place to start juicing for her. I was on a juice fast at the time, and was attempting to juice for both of us, which started to become a challenge. Luckily, it was brought to my attention, that rather than cutting up all the produce like I was doing, why not use my food processor's slicing mode to do the cutting for me. What a brilliant idea. "Thanks Louise!"

We started to look for another juicer, as we wanted it to be easy for my step-daughter to juice, once we...and my juicer, left to go back home.

I found an Aicok Juicer on Amazon for only $149. It had the single auger, masticating, slow juicer parts, but it also had a large chute, that has a slicer to cut the produce as it heads into the masticating section. Yes, the warranty is only two years, but it got her going at a great price.

You can spend anywhere from $150 and upwards to $2,595 on the one that the Gerson Clinic and Dr. Lorraine Day recommend. (Norwalk Juicer).

The best money that you will spend will be on your juicer. Look for one that has what is called a single auger, masticating, slow juicer. It crushes the produce, rather than spinning it, which allows you to do a slow juice (which preserves the nutrition) and is critical to be able to juice those nutrient rich greens! Also look for a 10 – 15-year warranty, so that you know the machine is sturdy for the amount of juicing that you are going to be doing.

In Canada the best place that I have found is on Amazon or Canadian Tire. In the USA, and other countries that are serviced by Amazon, I suggest that you start your search there. Again, I will put some links to great juicers on my website; ***www.AreYouinBalance.com***

Happy Juicing!

Basking in the Warmth

The first 'S' of the acronym, stands for Sunshine.

Nothing feels as good as the warmth of the sun upon your skin, especially after a long Canadian winter.

I would like to encourage you to not wait until summer, to savor the warmth of the sun. Start today!

The more days that you are able to get outside into the fresh air, and let the healing rays of the sun kiss your skin, the better.

Here are some of the benefits of the sun;
It eases stress and tension in your body
It elevates your mood
It renews your energy
It helps to normalize your thyroid hormone production
It increases the oxygen content of your blood
It kills germs

It helps improve your sleep patterns
It strengthens your immune system
It helps to reduce your cancer risk by producing natural occurring Vitamin D in your body

Just getting 30 minutes of sunlight onto your skin each day, has been shown to help prevent as well as reverse cancer in the body.

Unfortunately, we have been told that we need to protect our skin from sun exposure by slathering on toxin filled, sunscreen. We have been told that if we don't wear sunscreen, then we increase our risk of skin cancer. This could not be further from the truth.

Let me share a study with you.

Experimental animals were given ultraviolet light treatment for twenty-four weeks. Half of the animals were given a highly nutritious diet (the type you have hopefully changed to), and the other half were given the SAD diet. (the one that most North American's eat).

After twenty-four weeks, the animals were checked. The ones who were eating the Standard American Diet; 24% of them had developed skin cancer, whereas with the highly nutritious diet group; not one had developed skin cancer.

So, was it the sun exposure or the diet, that contributed to the skin cancer?

So why not just slather on sunscreen, just to be safe?

The majority of sunscreens are not something that you would be willing to eat due to all of the chemicals they consist of. If we are not willing to ingest it through our mouth, then in the light of desiring to not add more toxins to our system, I would like to remind you on what the largest organ of the body is... the skin.

You also want to absorb the Vitamin D, through your skin, as well as through your pupils, so expose as much of your skin as you can, as well as wear a hat or sun visor, rather than sunglasses. We need the brain to receive the sunlight, which it cannot do if the eyes are covered.

There is an exception to not wearing sunglasses. If you are skiing or boating, then because both snow as well as water reflect way too much sun, you need to wear sunglasses when out on a boat, or goggles in the case of skiing.

So, if you who are looking for a valid reason to go south for the winter, hopefully, I have now provided you with one. ☺

The Elixir of Life

The next letter in this acronym is 'W', which stands for Water.

How would you like to have beautiful skin, better mental clarity, more energy, assist your body in detoxifying, as well as replace what your body is usually crying out for?

This can all be done by drinking more quality water on a daily basis.

You see, our bodies are made up almost entirely of water. Our brain is 98% water. Our blood is 94% water. Our internal cell structure is 98% water, and as a whole, our body is 76% water.

Unfortunately, the majority of the population do not drink the amount of water needed to assist their body in removing the toxins that they are attempting to be broken down. We need to flush our insides with pure water.

I liken it to attempting to wash your car with a shot glass of water. How clean will it get? The only thing is, our health is far more sensitive to a lack of water, than our car is of being dirty.

I almost died from Heat Stroke when I was fifteen years old, from being out in the sun all day, and not drinking water. I lost my vision, as my body started to shut down. You can read the full story in my book, that will be released shortly after this one called; 'Where was God when I needed Him most?'

I chuckle inside when I have asked a client of how much water they drink on a daily basis, and receive the answer 'lots'. So, what is 'lots'? How much should you be drinking on a daily basis? Does coffee or tea count towards your daily needs?

If you have been diagnosed with cancer, you need a minimum of ten cups of water each and every day. I am not talking about beverages that you make with water, like coffee or green tea.

If you are still drinking coffee, then you need to understand that coffee is a diuretic, which means that it removes water from your body. For every cup of coffee or caffeinated tea, you drink, you need to drink an additional cup of water. By drinking coffee, you are also asking your pancreas to work extra hard. But please, if you are currently drinking more than a few cups of coffee a day, do not stop drinking it cold turkey. Instead, it is easier on you if you cut back one cup at a time, as you start to replace those cups of coffee with water.

If you are starting off with not drinking very much water, then start off at the amount of water you are currently drinking, and every 3 or 4 days increase it by another cup, until you are at your daily goal of water consumption.

You may be like a lot of people, including the way my husband use to be, having a hard time drinking enough water. No matter how much he knew that drinking water was good for his health, he just did not like the taste.

So, let's start there; the taste.

If you are drinking city water, then I do not blame you for not liking the taste. Chlorine and fluoride are not what I would consider pleasant to both the taste buds, nor to improving your health.

The National Cancer Institute found that drinking chlorinated water, increased the risk of developing bladder cancer. Chlorine also destroys vitamins A, B, C and E, as well as the feel-good amino acid tryptophan.

The VERY best water that you can drink is water freshly out of an artesian spring, as that is the way that God designed the water. It is non-chlorinated, non-fluoridated, full of minerals, naturally pH rich, and so refreshing.

When I was diagnosed with cancer as an adult, I was lucky enough to know a family who had discovered an artesian spring on their property, and was able to start drinking it.

You can ask around, or do a search in your area, to see if there is a local artesian spring that you can start getting water from.

If you cannot find one, then you may need to search out any of the options below. Keep in mind that the most important criteria is; that the water does not have chlorine or fluoride added to it, as these will work against your health.

a. Do you have a friend who has a well that gives them refreshing water? If you enjoy having a glass of water at their place, I am sure that they would be willing to help you with your recovery, by supplying you with jugs of water. You may need to go buy an empty jug, but that is a small price to pay for moving towards your healing.

b. If you do not have a friend who has quality water on their property, then search out bottled water. The preference is water that has not been 'de-mineralized', as this means that they have taken the alkalizing minerals out of the water, which the preference is to have the minerals left in. If that is all that you can find, then it is still way better to drink that, then city tap water.

c. You may be wondering about water machines that claim to raise the alkalinity of water. I have researched into them, and I am still not convinced either way on them. I know that they do make drinking the water so much easier. That is a good thing. My only concern is that you do not want to drink water that is much higher than 8.0 – 8.4 pH. So, as long as you do not think that the higher the alkalinity, the better, then if it gets you drinking more water, go for it. Personally, I would still look first for an artesian spring, as that is the VERY best.

Still not crazy about drinking water? Here are some options that helped my husband drink more water.

One way to make drinking water more pleasant while at the same time increasing your alkalinity is by added one of the following to your water; freshly squeezed lemon or lime, chlorophyll, chlorella, a bit of pure barley juice powder (if you are using it in all of your cups of water, then use it to just flavor the water or else you will detoxify too quickly).

If you have chosen to add lemon or lime to your drinking water, make sure that you buy the fresh fruit and squeeze out the juice. Even though the bottled lemon (Real Lemon is one brand), or lime may be easier to use, it does not have the same health principals. Freshly squeezed lemon juice will go bad in just a few days, even in the fridge. Why does the bottled ones, not go bad?

Another healthy option to improve the appeal of drinking more water, is adding a drop of either spearmint or lemon therapeutic essential oils. This is one time when convenience and health are found in the same bottle.

Before I leave the drinking water chapter, I need to tell you two more things.

First of all, it is imperative that for every ten cups of water that you drink, that you also consume (spread throughout the day), ¼ tsp of unrefined sea salt. Unrefined sea salt are ones like Himalayan Salt, or Redmond's Real Salt. They are naturally high in minerals, and have not been bleached as some sea salt have been. If it is pure white, then you know that it has been bleached, as sea salt is not pure white.

The reason for taking in a bit of sea salt spread throughout the day, is that as your body lets go of the water that you have taken in, your body will also be letting go of the critical minerals that keep your electrolytes balanced. Replacing these critical minerals, is easily done by sprinkling a bit of unrefined Sea Salt onto your food, or else into the palm of your hand, where you can just lick it.

The second thing is, if you currently weigh more than 160lbs, you may need to drink more than 10 cups of water each day.

To figure out how much water your particular body needs; take your current weight, and divide it in half. That is how many ounces per day you need to drink. If you take that number and divide it by 8 that is how many cups it equals.

Now that we have talked about drinking water, I will briefly remind you about the water you put onto your skin via a bath or shower.

When you have a shower or a bath, make sure that you are not introducing chlorine into your body through the hot water. Hot water opens the pours of your skin.

If you can, the best solution is to install a filtering system to your main water line, so that when you wash your hands, have a shower or a bath, you are not introducing chlorine into your body.

If this is not possible for you, either because you rent your place, or the cost is more than you are able to spend, then here are some other ideas of what I did.

If you like to have a bath, then I found an awesome solution. If you are a shower person, then there are lots of shower filters that you can hook onto your shower nozzle, including my favorite one. If you travel, the bath solution works well, as it is portable and does not require an attempt to travel with a wrench in your back pocket.

I found a product company called 'RainShowr', which has a solution for having a chlorine free bath, as well as an excellent shower filter. I take the 'RainShowr' bath ball with me when I travel, as it is totally portable.

Both the bath ball and the shower filter, work on a different premise than the filters that just attempt to block out the chlorine. What it does is that it converts the toxic chlorine into the non-toxic chloride. You will smell the difference right away. To make it easier for you to find, you can go to my website **www.AreYouinBalance.com**, where I share a link to it.

Lastly, if you like to swim in a swimming pool, then choose ones that use salt to sterilize rather than chlorine. This applies to hot tubs even more so, due to the water temperature opening up your skin pores. If you can, it is better to swim in the ocean, a river, or a clean lake. Ocean's and lakes have the extra bonus of providing you with the calmness of the water.

Taking Positive Steps Towards Recovery

Now for the 'E' in the acronym. It stands for Exercise.

Dr. Selye subjected 10 rats to stresses of light, noise, and electric shocks. In one month, all had died. Then he took 10 rats and subjected them to the same stresses, but also gave them exercise on a treadmill. After a month they were all well and thriving.

The conclusion: Exercise allows the body to make use of its restorative powers.

What are the best exercises to do? There are three different types of exercises; Cardiovascular, Stretches, and Strength building.

Walking as well as rebounding on a mini trampoline are the very best exercises for your heart, as well as your lymphatic system. Both have the ability to get your heart pumping, while jumping on a rebounder, is one of the few ways that you can open and close your lymphatic system.

Why would you care about opening and closing your lymphatic system? Unlike the heart, the lymphatic system does not have any type of pump to flush the toxins out, so not only does it aid in flushing out the toxins, it also flushes dead cells out of the body. It increases your red blood cell production, which is excellent to have lots of those.

It also has anti-inflammatory benefits. Do you remember me saying in the previous book, that inflammation is a contributor to developing cancer?

I was going to tell you all of the ways a rebounder helps you recover, but I found that it started to feel like information overload as I was writing them out for you. I promised at the beginning of this book that I would attempt to keep things as simple as possible, so let me put it this way; rebounding will benefit your immune system, your moods, and help your body to detoxify, as well as helps to increase your pH.

If you are unsteady on your feet, you can either buy a stabilizing bar for it, or else you can hold onto the back of a chair, when you are jumping. Eventually, your balance will improve and you will no longer need to hold onto anything.

A great DVD or book to read (later on), is called 'The Cancer Answer'. It is all about the research done on rebounding.

Strive to either walk for forty-five minutes each morning, or else rebound for fifteen minutes a day. Start where you are and gradually build up.

For strength building, body builders have discovered that rebounding seems to strength their muscles as well, as gravity provides resistance. The other option is to use exercise rubber bands, as they also provide the resistance needed.

For flexibility, doing stretches is the best way to achieve this. Stretches are an excellent way to end your day before heading to bed, as they tend to relax you as well.

Repair Work Underway

'R' in the acronym ANSWERS, represents the words Rest and Relaxation. This health principal is one that you cannot afford to skip over.

In order for your body to have the energy to do the repair work necessary, you need to give it lots of rest and relaxation. It is like asking a runner who just finished running a marathon, to go out dancing as he crosses the finish line. He just will not be able to do it. He is exhausted and needs to rest.

You may be a 'Type A' personality, where rest is not a part of your vocabulary. Both my husband and I are, so I fully understand. What about you, are you a 'Type A' personality? If so, it is even more important for you to stop working, in order to take your healing real serious. You need to focus on following all of the health principals.

It is very hard to make all the juices that you need to drink, and work at the same time. If you are a 'Type A' personality, put the same energy that you have put into your work, into your new position of doing what it takes for your body to heal.

I had a client who took a couple months off when she was first diagnosed with cancer. She faithfully followed what I had taught her, until her cancer appeared to be in remission. Then she returned to her stressful job, was unable to follow the full program, and started to eat the way she used to eat, once again. Her cancer returned, as she never did go back to what helped her in the first few months, as well as eating the foods that feed cancer. Sadly, I watched her pass away.

You may be saying; "I can't afford to stop working", or "We cannot afford for me to not work". Can I be REAL HONEST with you? If you do not stop working, your family will not only have the loss of your income forever, but they will have lost you as well.

Do whatever you need to do to facilitate putting your recovery as #1 priority. If you had a broken leg, or you just had open heart surgery, would you attempt to go to work?

The hardest part of developing cancer, is that often times, a person does not look like they are sick, (especially when you are following these health principals), so it is easy to forget, which is good for the mind, but not good for the 'doing part'.

When I was diagnosed, I had no energy to work. In fact, I barely had the energy to make my juices, but I knew that they were so important for my recovery. Unfortunately, once we arrived at the other side of the critical part of my healing with all the expenses we had incurred, along with me not being able to work, we had to declare bankruptcy. It was not what we wanted to do, but at the time, it was what was necessary. We have regained our good credit once again... and the most important part is that I am alive and well.

I know of someone who spent three hundred thousand dollars on their chemotherapy treatments, and they still died. On everything that we needed to buy, including going to the detox retreat, we spent less than five percent of that, so not only does the health rebuilding method cost much less than the medical method, but your chances of survival are so much higher.

Now that I have finished my lecture on not working, or worrying about the money, I will continue on.

Another real important habit that you need to get into, is going to bed by 9pm at the latest. Why do I say that? The hours between nine and midnight have the most restorative properties.

I was a night owl, so this was a hard adjustment for me. I am grateful that at the Detoxification Retreat, they physically shut off the lights at 9pm. By the time we went home again, both my husband as well as myself, were forming the new habit of going to bed by nine. So, if you are a die-hard night owl, YOU can do it. You may find at the beginning that because your circadian rhythms are so use to you being up late, that you cannot fall asleep right away, that's ok. You can either start going to bed one hour earlier than you currently are doing, and then after a few days go to bed another hour earlier, until you reach the goal of 9pm, or you can just jump in and go to bed at 9pm even if at the beginning you just lie there. It takes discipline, but your body will thank you for it.

If insomnia is an issue for you, I have found several things that have helped me.

Shut down being on the computer at least half an hour before 9pm.

Do something relaxing before going to bed. Stretches, or reading are good options.

Eat your last meal earlier in the day, rather than attempting to go to sleep on a full stomach.

If I am feeling really wound up or hyper, it is often due to my eating something that had MSG or wheat in it. So, I take a cup of water with activated charcoal in it, and go to bed. It works like a charm to absorb the toxins that are preventing me from sleeping.

Licking a bit of sea salt poured onto my hand just before going to bed, also helps, as it is loaded with minerals.

Magnesium and Potassium are minerals that relax the nervous system, so they can be helpful. There is a drink powder called Calm Magnesium, which if taken in hot water just before you go to bed, helps to relax you enough to fall asleep.

Vitamin B100 has helped me over the years as well. This is all of the B vitamins each having 100 mg, except the B12. For some reason, taking two B50's does not do the same thing. I found that the 'NOW' brand was excellent for this.

Some people find having a hot cup of herbal tea, helps them relax.

Soaking in a warm bath relaxes as well. Just make sure to have a glass of water if you have been perspiring while in the bath.

Going for a stroll in the evening, can be helpful. This is not your exercise walk, as you do not want to exercise before going to bed. This is just a relaxing walk where you take in the beauty all around you.

Doing deep breathing while lying in bed, helped me majorly when I first was having a challenge sleeping. You take in a deep breath through your nostrils, hold for a count of ten, and then let out through your mouth. Continue until either you fall asleep, or else you are fully relaxed. If you do it with your eyes closed, it relaxes you even more so.

The last health principal for having a great sleep, is to have fresh air coming into your bedroom while you are sleeping. Do you remember reading about that at the beginning of this section in the chapter called 'Breath of Life'?

So now, if you have ever wanted to find a good reason for sleeping in, or savoring the morning lying in bed, I hope that I have provided you a valid reason. It is not being lazy, it is good for your recovery!

Section 5
Healing Your Incredible Mind

No Hurry, No Worry

The last letter in the acronym 'ANSWERS', is another 'S', which is probably one of the most overlooked components to health; Stress Reduction. It is a huge factor affecting your immune system.

Back in 2005 when my chiropractor noticed the swelling in my lymph nodes, I was shocked when the diagnoses came back as Lymphoma. You see, I knew that I was eating pretty healthy. I walked every day. I got sunshine and fresh air pretty much every day. I drank lots of pure filtered water. I didn't drink or smoke, and basically led a healthy lifestyle. There was one lifestyle health principal though, where I was 'out of the ballpark'.

Stress was something that I had struggled with since I was in my teens. My stress was not acute, it was chronic. Acute stress we can easily identify, as it occurs during or shortly after a very stressful situation.

You may be like myself, and have taken tests to see how severe your stress is, and then the results stated that you did not have much stress, even though the reason you took the test in the first place, was because you suspected that stress was an issue for you. If they were asking questions about recently changing jobs, having a major loss of someone you love, or were having financial challenges, chances are that they are testing for acute stress. I always passed those with flying colors.

It wasn't until I stumbled upon a test that measured chronic stress, that my results came back; "get help immediately!" You see chronic stress does the most amount of damage to your immune system. It is like having your lights left on in your home 24/7. Eventually, the light bulb will burn out. Unlike a light bulb, the toll on your adrenals getting burned out, is far more serious.

Chronic stress is a major culprit behind both a person developing cancer, as well as hindering them from fully recovering. Unfortunately, chronic stress can sneak up on you. If you decide to join us for the online program, you will be given the opportunity to test how much chronic stress you are dealing with, and how it may be affecting your health.

Acute stress is not 100% harmless. I had a good friend who developed diabetes immediately after receiving some devastating news. Acute stress can switch to becoming chronic, by having numerous stressful situations, one after another in a short time span. Often you are not able to deal with the overload of emotions. So, we do need to protect ourselves from acute stress, if at all possible.

When I recognized that my cancer was brought on due to stress, I had no idea of how I could get rid of this chronic stress that I had been living with for so long. It had gotten to the point that it actually felt pretty normal.

I still remember to this day the moment I cried out to God; "How do I get rid of stress?"

My husband and I were camping at a very tranquil place, with the exception being that we were in both bear and cougar country. (You can read about that in my book, 'Where was God when I needed Him most?')

Camping amongst pine trees, and starting off my mornings sitting next to one of my favorite lakes on Vancouver Island, was awesome. Early in the morning, when most other campers were still sleeping, the lake was just like glass. I loved to sit and drink it all in, as it had a unique calming effect on my mind. Just thinking about it now, gives me a yearning to be there.

I remember one particular morning, that I was taking a walk through the woods. The birds were chirping. The sun was shining through the trees, and my mind went to the topic of stress. I cried out to the Lord asking him how to get rid of stress.

His answer was in the form of a picture in my mind. What I saw was one of those French soup bowls, that have a wide rim and are closer to the height of a salad plate, than a cereal bowl.

The bowl was full of steaming soup with a teaspoon next to the bowl rather than a regular soup spoon. Then I heard the whisper; "Savor Life".

I thought about it. When I eat soup with a soup spoon or a tablespoon, it is so easy to gulp down the soup, but if I eat it with a teaspoon, I can only consume a small amount at a time.

Like soup, when you take life in small amounts at a time, you actually have an opportunity to savor the journey, more so than if you either gulp down your soup, or run through life, without taking the time to fully take in all of life's experiences.

I remember once counselling a couple who were world class athletes. I was saddened as I listened to their pattern of what they would do after a race. Even when they won the race, which they usually did, they would not take time to savor the victory. Instead, as soon as the race was completed, they would focus their attention on their next race. How many of us do this exact same thing, with certain areas of our life? Are we so busy 'doing', that we forget to enjoy the journey?

One of the things that caught my attention in the small Mexican community that we lived in for almost half a year, was the attitude of the locals that we lived around. They had savoring life down to a fine art. They practiced a saying God had brought to my mind; "No Hurry, No Worry", as a part of their culture.

Coming from Canada where the culture of always being in a hurry, and the norm being worrying about something, or you are not considered normal; it took time to adjust to this new culture.

I found that it was a challenge for both me and my husband's 'Type A' personality to let go of our patterns from home, and start to adapt to the "No Hurry, No Worry" concept. Once I started to, my whole experience changed. I started to really savor the culture that I was surrounded with. I found myself smiling for no particular reason. I experienced a new type of happiness. It was a sense of internal joy. I never wanted to leave this culture and return to my 'always busy' life back in Canada.

Then, I realized that I could take the attitude home with me. I didn't have to follow the rest of the crowd. I could be a Maverick, and respond differently to the drive of always being in a hurry. Sometimes, we need to step out of the rat race, and reconsider what the hurry is all about. We also need to ask ourselves, will worrying about this situation, really change the outcome.

Yes, I could change the way I did things in any country of the world. It is just nice to surround ourselves with others who also, are not in a hurry, and have perfected the not worrying concept. I think that this will be a goal of the online program that I plan to offer. We can create our own mini 'Mexican culture' of supporting each other to practice the 'No Hurry, No Worry' lifestyle.

But you may be saying; "Donna, what about all those times that I have no control over the situation? What about when my husband drives me crazy? Or my kids continually fight with each other? Or I have a teenager, who is pushing my limits to the max? I am not in the 'Hurry Mode', nor am I in the 'Worry Mode'. How do I deal with those situations?"

You are absolutely right you may not be in the 'Hurry mode'... and you may be, without recognizing it. I will also challenge the thought that you are not in the 'Worry mode'. How can I say that? Are there teenagers in Mexico? Are there siblings there? Are there husbands? So, how can they still maintain their attitude?

You may need to ask yourself; "why am I getting upset right now? What is my fear? What is the REAL reason for my stress? Am I feeling out of control?"

If you are feeling out of control, what is the truth? Are these circumstances, actually something you have control over anyways? Who is the only one who can truly change the outcome of this situation?

I would like to invite you to give them all to Jesus. I am not talking about giving them to Him, and five minutes later, grabbing them back. Give them to Him and let Him handle the situation.

As hard as it may seem, Jesus loves your children even more than you could ever love them. He wants the very best for them, just like you do. He loves your husband too. He also wants YOU to be stress free. The only difference is that He has all of the answers on how to deal with things. He is far smarter than we are.

In the bible He encourages us to change knapsacks with Him. He will take our heavy load, in exchange for His empty knapsack. Go on, hand it over. He can deal with it. Let Jesus help you with what you have no control over anyways.

Looking for Beauty

Now we will look at the last three letters in the full acronym of 'pH.D. ANSWERS ABC'. The first letter of 'ABC' is of course 'A', which represents having an Attitude of Gratitude.

In the previous chapter called; 'No Hurry, No Worry', I was talking about my experience while living in Mexico.

One of the other things that I noticed while living there, was how they valued beauty. You saw it in how the women dressed. No matter how much they weighed, the women always looked attractive. The majority of women also wore makeup, or at least lipstick. Their traditional clothes and the color of their houses, also were vibrant. They LOVED beauty!

Despite how poor they were, the children were happy. They may have only one ball for all of the kids in the neighborhood to share, but they were grateful for that one ball. The parents were also happy, and would greet us with a genuine smile, when they invited us to come sit down so they could chat with us.

So, how could children without toys, as well as their parents all feel content in their poverty? They dwelt on what they did have, rather than what they didn't have.

I believe that it all has to do with our thinking. Are we grateful for what we do have, or are we focused on our losses?

Years ago, I acted in a play called 'Beauty through Spectacles'. In short, it was about a young girl, who saw beauty, where others saw a dreary world. Her secret, was some magical glasses that she found. She used these glasses to view the world around her. All she could see with these glasses on, was the beauty in people and her environment.

What about you? Do you have glasses on that serve your healing? Do you see the beauty, or do you need to switch your glasses, from ones that view the world as a negative, and harsh world? Are you viewing life as a blessing, or are you viewing it through negative thoughts? Are you thinking like a winner, or like a victim of your circumstances?

You see, whatever we look for, we will find.

As a counsellor of sexual abuse, I was awed at the difference between certain clients. Some who went through horrendous experiences, sometimes appeared to have suffered less trauma, compared to some clients who appeared to have experienced a relatively far lower amount of abuse.

How could that be? I found that it all had to do with how that particular person looked at life. Despite their experiences, some people still have a great attitude. It was because they did not consider themselves a victim, but a survivor. They did not allow the actions of others to define how they viewed themselves.

It is the same with surviving cancer. Those who view themselves as helpless or a victim of their diagnosis, will have a harder time getting well. That is why it is so important to be actively working on your healing process. When you are working on rebuilding your health, it gives you a sense of hope, purpose and control. You are in the driver's seat. It assists you on staying out of the victim ditch.

Those who go the medical route, can easily slip into the helpless ditch as the doctors take over, and their sense of control fades away. It is easy to feel like they no longer even have a say over their treatment protocol, or their own body. Unfortunately, feeling helpless or a victim, depletes our immune system even more so.

I want to encourage you to not slip into the helpless, negative, victim ditch. Instead, work towards being grateful for the measure of health that you do have, as you savor the beauty around you. Look for the beauty and you will find it. This attitude can only bless you and others.

Why not start a grateful journal! Each morning before you start your day, think about things that you are grateful for.

Are you grateful to have woken up this morning? None of us are guaranteed tomorrow. Are you grateful for having water to drink, or to be able to take a shower in?

My husband and I no longer take having water for granted. One morning when we awoke, we discovered when we went to flush the toilet and then wash our hands, that we had no water. What happened?

That particular night, the temperature had dropped so low that the water hose froze solid. You see we were living in our 5th wheel, and anxiously counting down the days until we closed down our home and headed to Mexico for the winter. Normally the temperature where we live, does not go down too low in the middle of October, but this night it did.

Luckily, the sun came out, and my husband was able to thaw the hose. We were so grateful to have running water once again.

You may wonder about our sanity when the very same thing happened the next night as well. Honestly, we just had so much on our mind, that we went to bed without considering that the weather forecast may not be accurate.

This time it was not as easy to rectify for two reason;

1. We needed to leave early in order to drive to the town that my husband was preaching in that morning.

2. The sun was not out in order to thaw the hose.

Luckily, we had another source of water to draw upon, that my husband could go fill up some jars with.

The next night… we ran water during the time that the temperature was dropping. We could hear the wind generators starting up on the surrounding farms, which signaled that the temperature was getting to a dangerously low number for the grapes and apples in our area.

So, what are you grateful for?

Getting Your Focus Off of 'Having Cancer'

This second to last letter, which is 'B', stands for Beyond Yourself.

When we are first diagnosed with cancer, it is very natural to be all absorbed with this life altering diagnose. Take the time to do that. Cry, get angry, question God... It is perfectly normal to go through a range of emotions, especially with this type of diagnoses.

I want to encourage you to grab a notebook or journal, and start writing all of what is going through your mind. I personally write to my Lord when I journal. I tell Him all that is on my mind; what I am happy about, what I am grateful for, what I am sad and what I am mad about.

I find it interesting to look back through what I wrote then, and how my prayer writing, has changed over the years.

That is the key; how it needs to change over time. Yes, it is perfectly fine to take the time to adjust to the news. At some point though, your focus needs to change. It needs to become 'other focused'.

What do I mean by 'other focused'? You need to start looking at how you can help others. How can you bless them? What prayer requests do they have?

Start praying for them. I have found that the more we look to see how we can bless others, that it improves our own well-being. I believe that this happens for two reasons;

1. God is always looking for reasons to bless us. As we pray for others, He lets it spill onto us as well.

2. Our mind is very powerful, and responds to what we tell it. It does not know if we are talking about ourselves or about someone else that we want to bless, so it blesses us as a bonus.

Unfortunately, the exact opposite will happen when we think or speak negatively about others. Again, our mind does not know if we are speaking or thinking negative thoughts about ourselves or someone else, so it will affect us negatively.

It has been shown that unforgiveness in our heart, will prevent a person from healing fully. It is like drinking a glass of poison, and expecting the other person to die. They may have long forgotten the incident(s), but if it is still affecting you, it needs to be addressed.

How do you know if it is still affecting you? Go off by yourself, and say out loud the person's name. Do you feel any part of your body tense up? Do you get a knot in your stomach, or feel tension in your jaw? Do you feel tension in your chest, or do you feel your hands tightening up? Chances are that if you felt any of the above symptoms, that something that they did, or said to you, is still affecting you.

Another way to test if they are still affecting you, is if you have a blood pressure monitor. Test to see what happens to your blood pressure when you say their name.

Right now, you may be feeling resistant to even the thought of forgiving this particular person. I have heard people over the years say; "I will never forgive ________ for as long as I live!" Why shorten your lifespan over something they have done or said to you? Yes, what they did was horrible! But you are the one who lose out if you hold onto resentment and ill feelings.

Let's first of all dispel some myths about forgiveness.

Forgiving someone, does not mean that what they did to you, was OK.

It does not mean that you need to have a relationship with them after forgiving them.

Forgive and forget are not part of the same equation. Remembering may be good for your safety.

It does not mean that the person does not need to suffer the consequences of their actions.

Forgiving someone does not mean that you are weak. It means that you are courageous.

The person does not need to ask for you to forgive them in order for you to.

The person does not need to even know that you have forgiven them. In fact, you can forgive people who are no longer alive.

So how do you forgive someone? You become curious about what was going on for them at the time they said the hurtful thing. You can become curious about their upbringing, and what trauma's they went through, to inflict pain on someone else. You recognize that hurting people, hurt other people.

One day I was chatting with a psychologist who ran therapy groups for men who were in prison for sexual assault. I asked him, a question that I had been pondering. I asked him of all the men that he worked with, who had sexually assaulted someone, how many had also been sexually abused themselves. He stopped to reflect on my question, then he answered... "All"!

You see emotionally, whole and healthy people do not intentionally hurt others.

By becoming curious about the person who has hurt you, it is impossible to feel anger at the same time. By becoming curious, you start to develop empathy for that person. Empathy is where 'the sting' falls away. Why? Because you are no longer focusing on 'what they did to me'. You are instead focusing on the pain of someone other than yourself.

There is another person that you may need to forgive in order to turn your health around.

Yourself!

Have you 'beaten yourself up', over things that you have previously done? Have you forgiven yourself for being a human being? Guilt weighs us down emotionally. Our emotions affect our physical well-being.

If you have hurt someone by your actions, have you considered taking it to God and ask Him to also forgive you? He doesn't have a big stick, just waiting to smack you. He wants us to come to Him. He wants to comfort us. He knows that unforgiveness of others or ourselves, hurt our immune system. He is there for you to talk to.

Cultivating Your Sense of Humor

A merry heart doeth good like a medicine
Proverbs 17:22

The very last letter, but definitely as important as the other eleven, is 'C', which represents Comical.

Have you ever watched the movie 'Patch Adams'? It is one of my favorite Robin Williams movies.

In case you have not seen it, it is about a guy who wants to become a doctor, but sees a huge hole in the medical system. He sets out to bring joy and laughter to the patients in the hospital that he is doing his intern in, much to the disapproval of the head dean of his medical school. The movie itself is hilarious, as you watch the way that Robin Williams goes about attempting to change the way things are done when it comes to patient care. This movie displays an excellent example of how healing, laughter can be.

We both know that being diagnosed with cancer is no laughing matter, so I will not attempt to downplay it. What I really want to encourage you to do, is to embrace the truth behind Proverbs 17:22.

Do you currently have a merry heart? If Yes, that is great. If no, then this is an area that you need to work on. Cultivate your sense of humor.

I don't know about you, but I have found that when I no longer find things funny, that I use to laugh at, it signals to me that things need to change. It is my mini barometer. I know that I am depressed when I no longer see the lighter side in life.

So how can you either maintain or regain your sense of humor?

When I first was diagnosed, some of my old favorite TV shows that as a teenager I would laugh at, like Gilligan's Island, I no longer found funny. So, I kept on searching, and discovered that I still found 'I Love Lucy', extremely funny, so I invested in every one of her videos that I could get my hands on. I then started to watch them on a daily basis. I was very purposeful on having laughter as part of my health regime. But eventually a person can run out of episodes to watch, so then what?

Watching funny shows or movies, is a great way to kickstart your sense of humor, but you want to eventually graduate to having an inner sense of joy and light heartedness. You want to be able to cultivate your OWN sense of humor.

If your sense of humor has left you completely, like mine had, start by watching things that you find funny. Even if you currently have your sense of humor, why not make an emergency list of different comedians that you find funny.

A great Christian comedian is Chonda Pierce. I like that there is no swearing or other offensive material in her presentations. My husband recently found a comedian on YouTube that we both find funny. Her name is Jeanne Robertson. Again, she does not swear either.

If you need to redevelop your laughing muscles, then start with being passively entertained. Next, you need to start working on your inner joy.

I remember when we had a pastor, whom we called Pastor Mike. I loved to be in his bible studies as his extremely subtle sense of humor, I found emotionally uplifting. I knew that in order for me to burst out in a hearty chuckle, in a bible study, my sense of humor was very much primed. I had so much inner joy at the time, that it was easy for me to see life on a lighter side.

What about you? Do you feel like you are under a dark cloud, or do have your sense of humor still intact?

You may be wondering how you go about cultivating an inner sense of humor, especially for those times that you have no internet access.

Do you remember in the 'No Hurry, No Worry' chapter, I talked about having discovered myself smiling for no particular reason, and having an inner joy? It is easier to cultivate your sense of humor, when you are not stressed out. Stress is a wet blanket on our sense of humor.

In the last two chapters before this one; 'Getting your Focus off of Having Cancer', as well as 'Looking for Beauty', helps prepare your mind to see the comedy in a situation.

When we forgive others, as well as focusing on other people, rather than on our current situation, when we look for and appreciate the beauty all around us, we naturally have a huge burden lifted off of us. When we no longer are under the weight of this type of heavy load, it is far easier to smile.

So... How's your sense of humor doing? If it is not up to snuff, you may find it helpful to start by watching comedians. Then go back and review the previous chapters in this section. It is also totally ok to take notes to create your own private blueprint on how you are going to 're-find' your sense of humor. This is too important to just skim over.

Section 6
Pulling it All Together

Where Do I Start?!!!

You may be feeling overwhelmed right now, wondering where do you start?

Depending on your personality and how aggressive your cancer is, you can either take one step. Have it become a part of your daily routine, and then add in the next step. Or you may want to add in one or two new steps every 2nd day.

If you are Stage 1 or 2, you have the luxury of choosing which method works best for you.

If you have been diagnosed with Stage 3 or 4, you will need to add in each step as quickly as you can. You cannot play with this, to 'see if it works'. You need to take your recovery very seriously. This needs to become your fulltime job.

If you are stage 4, I personally would go to the Gerson Clinic or Hippocrates Institute, as they can help you start reversing it very quickly. If you just cannot come up with the money, no matter how hard you try, either look for less expensive detox retreats, or find a health coach or someone who will support you to follow ALL of the health principals we have gone over, each and every day.

Support is so important to your recovery. If you find that you need additional support, I suggest that you consider joining my online education and support program. There, you will be supported on following all of the health principals that you have been reading about, at a fraction of the cost. I hope this will help you to be able to afford it.

No human can tell you which way is the best way for you to approach your healing journey, but from my own personal experience, following is the order that I would do.

If you are a Christian start by praying and asking God to guide you on your journey. If you are not a Christian, that's ok God still would love to hear from you, but He never forces anyone to chat.

Next, get yourself some activated charcoal powder. You can go to the internet to locate it. Just make sure that it is a fine powder, rather than the capsules, and buy it in a canister rather than a bag. Believe me, you will be happy that you did, as the powder is so fine, that in a bag, you can easily stain your clothes and counter tops.

Until you are out of the critical zone, you need to give your body every opportunity to heal, by avoid adding more toxins into your body.

Start with cutting out the three food items that feed cancer the most; cheese (and other dairy products), sugar, and wheat.

Buy yourself a juicer and start drinking some homemade juices.

Increase your juices until you are drinking between ten and thirteen cups per day. Personally, you may want to consider immediately starting a sixty-day juice fast.

When you go back onto food after the sixty days, then I would eat 100% organic, raw fruits and vegetables, along with continuing your thirteen juices. By doing 100% raw and organic, your pH will be brought into the balance quicker than if you do seventy-five or eighty percent raw.

If you are stage 1 or 2, and you are not mentally ready to start a juice fast by itself, then for your meals, include raw fresh vegetables and some fruit especially lemons, grapefruits, apples, blueberries and other berries.

Go for a walk each morning, and if you have a rebounder start jumping a few minutes each day. Slowly increase the jumping until you are jumping for fifteen minutes.

Take in some deep breaths of fresh air, and keep a window open at least a few inches while you sleep at night.

Aim to get to bed by 9pm each night.

Increase your water consumption until you are drinking a minimum of ten cups per day.

Start to do a detox program, either at a retreat or at home.

Watch or read something funny each day.

Work on forgiving all those who have hurt you.

Actively look for ways to unwind, that works for you

Don't sweat the small stuff. Let go of "it's not fair"

Start a grateful journal

Look for ways to be a blessing to others

What About Herbs & Supplements?

There are some wonderful herbs and supplements that can assist you on your journey. Yes, some of them even are known to cure cancer. The only trouble with viewing them as your answer for getting well, is that you did not develop cancer from a lack of these herbs or supplements. So, if you do not do anything different with your lifestyle, after reading the proceeding chapters, does it make sense to you that the cancer would return?

I cannot emphasize this too strongly; use the herbs and/or supplements as an EXTRA to get you back on your feet again but make a commitment to follow the lifestyle changes for the rest of your life.

If you choose to use herbs, make sure that you get them from a reliable source. If the potency is not there, then you are wasting your money as well as precious time taking something that is not giving you the results.

One of the criteria that I use to examine a product, is I look into the company and look to see why the company was started. Was it started because the founders had a personal experience and wanted to share it with others, or are they just business minded and saw a market they wanted to tap into?

Two years after I was told that I had Lymphoma, I was introduced to a company called Nature's Sunshine Products. I looked into it carefully and found that the founders of the company had a health issue that cleared up from herbs and wanted to share it with others. I was impressed that they had been around since 1972 and that as a Natural Health Consultant with a lot of knowledge about the value of certain herbs, I could buy individual herbs as well as combination ones at a reasonable price, for my clients. I was especially happy that their detoxification herbal combination was what I would have put together myself.

Lastly, they not only had extreme high standards for the quality of their herbs, but they also treated their consultants with respect and care. They even had partnered with a wonderful school to educate their consultants in how to use which herbs and when.

So yes, I am bias in where I buy my herbs, but you need to determine where you get yours from. All of the HERBS listed below, I can help you obtain at wholesale prices.

If you would like to set up an account in order to get them at my discount, you can go to

http://HelloHealth.mynsp.com, choose your country, and set up an account for yourself. The other option is, you can send me a private message through Messenger, and I will help you set up an account in your country. You can find me on Facebook and Messenger under Donna Marie Hockley. I am the maverick wearing the black cowboy hat.

Some people wonder why I want to help you get them at my cost, rather than trying to make a profit off of it. It is because I want to help you get what you need at the best price. You have enough other expenses to deal with, without supplements adding to the mix. (...and even more so, if you need Paw Paw because you did Chemo before you knew not to)

Below are the herbs and supplements that I believe are helpful.

Paw Paw (Asimina triloba), is a 'natural' chemo therapy. It will not destroy your healthy cells but will kill the cancer cells. It does this by cutting off the blood supply to the cancer cells. If you have already done chemotherapy, please read the chapter; 'But I already did chemotherapy', in my first book. It is imperative that you use this herb to help offset the chemotherapy resistant cells that would have been created.

This herb is not a preventative one. It is not meant to help prevent you from developing cancer in the first place. It only helps to destroy cancer cells that are already there.

It can be used in conjunction with chemo therapy if you choose that route. Most doctors will not want you to use it while you are having chemotherapy because it does lessen the side effects that they are monitoring, so it confuses them.

Always keep in mind that it is your body and you are the only one who can choose what you will go with, for your recovery protocol.

It is important to know that yes, it is from the Gravolia plant family, but true North American Paw Paw (Asimina triloba) has been shown to be 24 - 50 times more potent than Gravolia itself.

Unfortunately, some companies are calling Graviola "Brazilian Paw Paw", but again this is not the true Paw Paw that you want for the potency. Other names for graviola are custard apple, cherimoya, guanabana and soursop. I enjoyed eating the soursop fruit while in Mexico, but please do not rely on these alternate ones as a potent cancer treatment.

For a lot more information about Paw Paw, you can do one of two things;

1. You could do a search online for Dr Gerry McLaughlin and Paw Paw, as he was the scientist who discovered the benefits of it. Here is one link; **http://www.pawpawresearch.com/graviola-inferior.html**

2. Or a friend of mine wrote an excellent book called "The Paw Paw Program - A 'Christopher Columbus' Approach to Cancer". You can find it by going to my website **www.AreYouinBalance.com**

Pau D'Arco (also known as Taheebo) works well with Paw Paw on cancer. It can also be used without Paw Paw. In fact, there is a doctor who has been reversing cancer with this herb alone, but it is important to take the same dosage as he gives his patients.

It assists the body in detoxifying. Candida, bacteria, fungus, viruses and parasites are destroyed with this particular herb. It also helps with inflammation, is a blood purifier and builds up the immune system.

Do any of these benefits sound familiar? They address a large amount of the root causes of cancer. It is also one of the Evergreen Trees.

Pau D'Arco can be used even when you do not have cancer. As I say above, it is great to help your body detoxify. I would use it a few times a year as part of your regular detoxification regime.

For people who choose chemotherapy, it helps with the side effects, as it is removing the toxins that are being injected into you. I personally question if I would spend money on chemotherapy and then remove it. I would just work on removing the toxins that caused the cancer with this and other herbs. Again, only you can decide on what you feel the most comfortable doing.

Warning: Pau D'Arco is a blood thinner, so it is not a good idea to use it if you are about to have surgery, or if you are using Warafin which also thins the blood.

E-Tea is the original formulation of Essiac Tea. When I looked at the ingredients, I could see why Rene Caisse helped so many people with this native formulation. All of the plants are very alkalizing to the body, thus raising the pH. They also help the blood, lymphatic system and liver to detoxify. Essiac tea does not work on the tumor itself. It is a cleanser, and stimulates the immune system. Like other beliefs of the Native culture, where this formulation originally came from, it addresses the root cause of the cancer developing. It improves the environment of your cells, so it can also be used as a yearly preventative.

For cancer, it is recommended that you take it as a tea. If you occasionally need it to be more portable, you can take the capsules with warm water.

CAUTION: If you have a brain tumor, this herbal combination is NOT advisable, as part of the healing process from these herbs, may expand the tumor 1st, before it starts to break the tumor down. This could cause pressure put onto a blood vessel. Not a good idea for the brain area.

Essential Liquid Minerals Minerals are CRITICAL for assisting the body to get into pH balance. When I first started taking the Essential Liquid Minerals, it seemed like I could not get enough of it and was counting down the hours until I could take another tablespoon. Then I found out that it is perfectly fine to take as much as your body is wanting for short periods of time.

Chinese Liquid Chi Tonic is an awesome combination of Chinese herbs that quickly repairs your adrenal system. If you have been under a lot of stress, chances are that your adrenals are in crisis. One symptom of your adrenals needing help, is extremely low energy. Taking a couple of ounces of this a day, cannot do you any harm, and you may be pleasantly surprised of how much better you start to feel.

Warning: it doesn't taste very good, but it sure makes you 'light up' with energy.

HSN-W are minerals from whole food sources, rather than from isolated chemically produced. This is the way that the body can recognize the minerals the best. (and vitamins for that matter).

These herbs are also great for the immune system, the glandular system, the thyroid, nerves, anxiety, skin, bones, arthritis and a lot more. I find that they really help me have a good sleep if I take one just before going to bed.

Red Clover is an incredible blood cleanser. It is said that life is in the blood, and I truly believe that our blood could always use an extra boost in cleansing it.

Warning: If you have an estrogen positive breast cancer, I would seek out a Natural Health Practitioner before adding this into your protocol, as there is controversy about the use of it if a woman's breast cancer is estrogen positive.

The same applies if you are currently taking Warfarin. If you are not using Warfarin, nor have an estrogen positive breast cancer, then this is an excellent blood cleanser. For those who cannot use Red Clover, remember that E-Tea also cleanses your blood.

Proteas Plus is a specific probiotic that if you take it on any empty stomach, between meals, it assists breaking down the shell around tumors, so that it is easier to be destroyed.

Cat's Claw Combination is also known as Una de Gato in Spanish. It is one of the Amazon's most impressive traditional healing herbs, as well as being a great support for the immune system. They combine it with the benefits of Astragalus as well as Echinacea. You now have a powerhouse of immune support.

Two of the three ingredients (Cat's Claw, and Echinacea) MAY interfere with Warfarin. I have a client who has not had any issues with it, but if you are taking this blood thinner, I would encourage you to work with a Naturopath to monitor your progress.

Astragalus the last individual product that I would like to suggest to start off with, not only is good for cancer as it helps to activate the T Cells and the Natural Killer cells, it also builds up the immune system. If you are taking Warfarin, this is a safe alternative to using the Cat's Claw. If you have Diabetes or Lupus, it is also good for that. You may wonder if it builds up the immune system, then wouldn't it be not good for an autoimmune disease like

Lupus. Unlike herbs that stimulate the immune system, Astragalus works by balancing the immune system.

I hope that the above list of these herbs, will help you if you were questioning what else can you do in ADDITION to the twelve lifestyle principals that we looked at. They are not a replacement for the lifestyle principals, but especially if you are currently in Stage 3 or 4, or if you have already done chemotherapy, they can help you 'get out of a pickle' that you have found yourself in.

What Else Can I Read or Watch?

I would like to encourage you to read, watch DVD's and search out additional information, based on the Truth!

Listed below are books, DVD's and Websites, that I especially would like to recommend for further study on your own.

Books I recommend:

'Cancer Step Outside the Box', 6th Edition, Bollinger, Ty (2014)

'Fresh Vegetable and Fruit Juices what's missing in your body, Walker', Norman. W (1979) Norwalk Press

'Juicing for Life', Calbom, Cherie and Keane, Maureen (1992) Avery Books a division of Penguin Group

'The Battle for Your Health Is Over pH', Gary Tunsky, (2006) Crusader Enterprises

'The Gerson Therapy', Gerson, Charlotte and Walker, Morton (2006) Kensington Books

'The Paw Paw Program - A "Christopher Columbus" Approach to Cancer', Loraine Benoit

'Your Body's Many Cries for Water', Batmanghelidj, F. (1995) Global Health Solutions, Inc

'Chris Beat Cancer: A Comprehensive Plan for Healing Naturally', Chris Wark (2018) Hay House Inc

And... of course the 'Bible'

DVD's I recommend:

'A Beautiful Cure'

'Cancer Doesn't Scare Me Anymore', Dr. Lorraine Day

'Fat Sick and Nearly Dead', Joe Cross

'He Loves Me, He Loves Me Not', Dr. Lorraine Day

'The Beautiful Truth', Steve Kroschel and Mike Anderson

'The Gerson Miracle', Steve Kroschel

'Healing from the Inside Out', Mike Anderson,

'The Cure for Cancer... Continues'

'Forks over Knives', Brian Wendel, Dr. Colin Campbell, and Dr. Calwell Esselstyn

Websites I recommend:

www.ChrisBeatCancer.com

www.thetruthaboutcancer.com

www.gerson.org

www.gersontreatment.com

www.GoodbyeCancerHelloHealth.com

www.DonnaMarieHockley.com

www.AreYouinBalance.com

https://www.youtube.com/watch?v=Sv8ACLTeEHE

Section 7
Up Close and Personal

My Own Struggles

Have you ever gone to the fair and wandered through the game booths?

There is one particular game that most closely resembles my struggles. It is the gopher one, or as my fourteen-year-old illustrator correctly calls it; 'Whac-a-mole'.

If you are not familiar with it; you are given a Styrofoam bat, and the objective of the game, is that as the gopher/mole pops up his head through one of the holes, you bat it down, before the gopher goes down the hole once more. Then another one pops up through another hole, and you need to quickly bat him down as well.

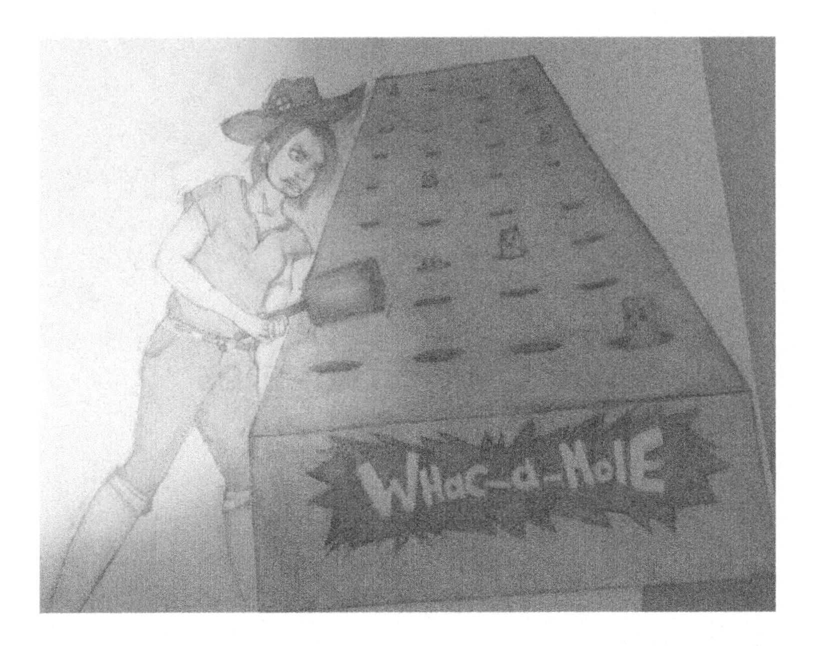

How was this like my life? The board was like my life as a whole. Each of the holes, that the gophers could pop up through, was representing one of the health principals that I had been endeavoring to do...in my own strength of course.

When the gopher pops up his head, and I try to bat it down, is how out of control that I was feeling. I may master one health principal, but then I started neglecting another one. So then, I would focus on that one, and start neglecting another one.

My relationship with God was radically altered one morning, while I was on my morning walk. This particular day, my walking partner was not available, so I went by myself.

It was a beautiful, sunny, but still crisp spring morning, and the tranquility was awesome. Sometimes God needs to get us alone, in order to really talk to us. This was one of those times.

He and I were talking about all twelve of the health principals that I outlined in Section 2 called 'The Whole Enchilada'. I was expressing my frustration on not being able to consistently do each and every one of them.

The Gopher game came as a full panoramic view in my mind as I cried out; "I can't do it!!!" I was in tears, as I desperately wanted to do all that God had taught me about the health building principals.

It was like I heard Him say to me; "Finally! You are right, you cannot do them all in your own strength".

The tears flooded down my cheeks, as I came to the realization that this was not something that I could just try harder, or grit my teeth and be able to remain in control.

I had always prided myself with embracing the saying; "If it is to be, it is up to me". But this was not God's desire for me. He wanted me to not rely on myself, but to let go and give Him the control of my life.

I needed to come to the realization, "that if it was to be, it was up to Him". I had to come to the place that even if I died, that was up to His plans, not mine.

I don't know if you are a control freak like I am, but if you happen to be a 'take charge' type of person, and not achieving what you set out to do, not being part of your thinking process, I want to encourage you to allow the Holy Spirit to talk to you right now.

You see, there can only be ONE King on the throne. It is either God or it is us. (Hopefully you have not put a doctor or a pastor into that position on the throne.)

I had to come to the place, where I could see my weakness... Did I just say that? I had to recognize how I was not capable of healing myself. Over and over again, I had failed miserably with my attempts to do it in my own strength.

Then a very foreign concept came to my mind. God did not NEED me to do the health principals in order to heal me. He could heal me instantly if He thought that was the best option for my personality, and circumstances.

He knows that for some of us, if He instantly healed us, we would not work on changing our bad lifestyle habits, that broke down our immune system in the first place. It would not be very long, before our body would develop cancer all over again.

What type of testimonial would that be to the world, if God instantly healed us of cancer, and then six months, a year, two or even five years later, we developed cancer all over again? What would non-believers, and even some professed Christians say about God and His lack of power to truly heal us? God's name would not be honored. In fact, the opposite would happen. Non-believers would not be drawn to want to know this wonderful God that we know. They would inaccurately think that God was somehow not strong enough to heal us 'for good'.

Unfortunately, the truth would not be seen. That yes, God did heal us, AND we had repeated what caused our body to develop cancer in the first place.

I liken it to our life being like a gigantic puzzle, and God has all of the pieces to the puzzle. He also has the box. We can only see our small little part, where we currently are. But God has our whole life mapped out.

So, what God taught me, was that no, He didn't need me to do the health principals in order to heal me. I needed to do the health principals out of my love for Him and to honor His name. I needed to get into the habit of honoring this body that He created. That this body did not belong to me, as He bought it with His blood.

I needed to come to the place where I finally gave up on trying to get well. I had to let go, and get myself out of the way. I had to finally come to the place where I admitted that I could not get well in my own strength. That I did not have any will power over appetite in my own strength. That sugar and cheese still called my name. I had to embrace "With man this is impossible. But with God ALL things are possible".

God wants to be the ruler of our life, but He is too much of a gentleman, to force His way there.

I have discovered that this journey is not a smooth, straight path. Our emotions can, and do go all over the place.

When I was first diagnosed, I seemed to be fine with the diagnosis. My family and friends were another story. They appeared to have a much harder time with it than I did. They seemed to be grieving before I even died, with the thought of losing me to this 'inevitable death sentence'.

My husband would pull-over to the side of the road and just weep in private. He thought that he needed to put on a strong front for me, so he held it together until he was alone.

Maybe I was in denial, or maybe it just hadn't sunk in as yet, but I was not afraid at all…at the beginning. I was extremely optimistic that I was not going to die. I believed that I just needed to follow the health principals that I already knew, and learn what I may not know as yet, from those who had also gone the natural route and lived.

I was fortunate to have a very positive Naturopath, who told me at each appointment, that I was not going to die. His demeanor was a calm and an assuring one, which helped me block out all of the fear that I was being bombarded with, from the outside world.

Then friends who were diagnosed close to the same time as myself, but who went the medical route, started to die. It seemed that people were dying from cancer, all around me.

Reality seemed to hit! My faith began to waver. I took my eyes off of the true Physician and started to focus on my own weakness. I knew in my heart that I was not doing all that I knew to do. I knew that I was not drinking all thirteen juices. My weight was going up, higher than I had ever weighed in my life... even when I had been pregnant. I started to question if I would also die.

I dropped into a depression, as I faced the possibility that maybe I would not live. The words to a song by Tim McGraw, called "Live like you're dying", played over and over again through my mind. Previously, I had embraced the words that described truly 'living'. But now, my mind went to the dying aspect.

I had no-one that I felt like I could talk to about what I was going through. I didn't want to upset my husband. I certainly didn't want to talk to my friends who already had a hard time with my decision to reject the medical model.

I didn't need their well-meaning pressure to reconsider what I was doing. I just needed a safe place to talk to others or even just one other person, who knew what I was going through because of their own journey with cancer. Unfortunately, I didn't know anyone else at that point in time who was going 100% the natural route, that I could talk to.

I started questioning in my mind, what I needed for this phase of my life? Many people when they and their loved ones believe that they are going to die, they attempt to fulfill the items on their bucket list. It might be a trip to

Hawaii, or to go in a hot air balloon, or to just to be surrounded with their loved ones.

Color is something that is extremely important to me. It can nourish my soul, and provide tranquility for me. It can alter my mood.

I didn't want to go anywhere. I didn't have the energy to go anywhere! But I wanted to alter my surroundings, so I hired a painter. I had her come in and paint my bedroom a beautiful color. A color that I would like to spend my last days in. The room felt peaceful to me. I was preparing myself mentally to die.

Sometimes we just need a safe place to talk about what we are going through. There is comfort in confiding in someone who truly understands because they have walked a similar journey.

I got through this hard time by talking to God. I journaled to Him everything that I was going through. I was brutally honest with all of my thoughts and feelings. I knew that He would not be horrified to hear what I was going through. I knew that He was there for me 24/7.

Support, Support, Support

Dear Family and Friends of the reader of this book

I do not know if you are a spouse, child, parent, friend or a relative of someone who has developed cancer. That part is not important. What I share with you will apply no matter what your relationship is.

I personally assume that the reason that you are reading this chapter, is that you care very much for the wellbeing of your loved one.

I am sharing this part with you so that you might know how to best support this person whom you desire to see make it through this journey.

I hope you don't mind me being straight forward when I write to you. Your support, can make a huge difference in their chance of survival.

So how do you support your loved one?

Only they can tell you 100% of what they need from you. Encourage them to be honest with you, of what would be most helpful. Remind them that it is not being selfish to ask for what they need.

I am guessing that the best gift they could ever give you, is to live. So, by them communicating what they need, enables you to support them in giving you and your family this precious gift, of surviving.

Whatever they say is the most helpful, may be what they need right now. That can change, as they progress through their own emotional journey.

Be patient with them, as stress will only hinder their recovery.

Know that your support is so appreciated, even if they do not have the emotional strength to express this to you. I know that sometimes, I felt like I was holding onto sanity with my fingertips, and zero ability to give back to others.

Some practical ways to support

Until your loved one, starts to recover, expect their energy to be low. They are not being lazy. Their body is doing all that it can to hold onto life.

The fastest energy booster is those 13 juices. I know that there have been times when I have felt like I was dragging myself along, and I was desperate for a revitalizing juice.

It becomes a vicious cycle of not having the energy to do what I knew would make me feel better. I needed the juices to have energy, but I needed energy to make the juices.

So, make their 13 juices for them each day. The biggest hindrance to drinking them on a regular basis is the chore of making them.

Often you will have people ask what they can do to help. If you cannot make the juices yourself, because your work schedule prevents it, then ask someone who has volunteered, to come help you do it for your loved one. Better yet, have a few different people take turns on coming over to make the juice. You could even have someone share the load with you making them.

If you do not have anyone that you can ask to make the juices, then hire someone. It is well worth the money to have a person come in for an hour or two each day, to provide life giving nutrients to your loved one.

I had a girlfriend who asked me what she could do to help me, when I was diagnosed with cancer. I asked her to scrub my carrots, and then bag them in large Ziplock bags for me. This was a great help as it eliminated one whole step for my juicing.

Go on a cleanse with them. If you can afford it, both of you go do the detox retreat. I felt so supported when my husband came with me, and then we followed up with a healthy eating pattern when we got home. The benefit that he got, was that he lost excess body fat that he had been carrying around with him, and had more energy than previously. The benefit that I received was feeling supported, and being able to share this part of my recovery with my husband.

Eat the foods that they need to eat in order to get well. Familiarize yourself in what foods nourish the body and which will hinder their recovery.

Don't bring junk food into the house. Avoid eating things that feed cancer, anywhere around them.

The truth of the matter is, the chance of you developing cancer or some other life-threatening disease is higher than the general population. The reason for this is due to the stress a person goes through with the prospect of their loved one dying. This is the time that YOU need to put high nutritional food into your body as well. You need to fortify your immune system to withstand the stress you are facing.

If you have young kids, take them out so that the person can rest or even sleep.

Go for a walk with them in the evening, so that they can unwind before they head to bed.

Do not question why they need to do all 12 heath principals outlined in this book. The last thing they need, is to argue over something that they are just starting to do.

Try to do as many of the health principals with them, as you can. This says support like nothing else does. Plus, as

I indicated earlier, you need to work on preventing this from taking a toll on your own health.

Emotional Support is sooooo important. I was extremely grateful that my husband stood behind my conviction to go the natural route.

If you are not convinced that it is the right choice for your loved one, educate yourself, by reading my first book; 'What You *NEED* to Know To Survive Cancer.' Maybe even check out some of the resources that I have provided at the end of section six. Watch them together. I was extremely grateful that my husband watched the videos with me.

They DO NEED a juicer, so support them in purchasing the type I recommend, as it will not only save money on the amount of produce needed, but it will also give them more nutrients with each cup of juice. I had to learn this the hard way.

Take them out into nature as often as you can. Go for walks in the forest, or if they enjoy camping, take them camping... just the two of you.

If they were working when they discovered that they had developed cancer, they NEED to stop working in order to focus on getting well. Support them on doing this. If it means that you now need to go to work, do it. If it means that you as a family need to cut back on expenses, as you downscale to a one income household, do it. Take the pressure and guilt off of them not providing the income for the family right now.

Some people say; "but we can't afford them to not work". Honestly, if they do not take the time to recover fully, you will lose way more than their contributing income. Yes, it may even mean that you have to declare bankruptcy, if you cannot handle your debt load without their income. Just do whatever it takes to support them on their journey to move from cancer, back into health.

Don't let money be a deciding factor on any of your choices, especially when it comes to things like a quality juicer, fresh organic produce (if you cannot grow your own), help around the house, Paw Paw if they unfortunately did chemo, and especially them taking a leave of absence from working, for at least a year after they are fully recovered. If they were stage three or four, they will need to take two years off from work, and continue doing all of the 12 areas for those two years.

Money problems, is the least of your worries. You can always regain your credit score, but you cannot bring them back, if they jeopardize their healing process.

If you would like to talk to other people who are supporting loved ones, I provide a private online support group that is specifically for the Support Person. It is a private place that you can be honest about what YOU are going through. It is a place for you to download without adding more burden to your loved one, with others who are going through what you are going through. It is a free bonus with the online educational/ support program that I offer.

Other People Did It, So Can YOU!

I hesitated on labeling the following testimonials by the 'type' of cancer that the person was told that they had. The reason that I questioned if I wanted to, was because of my understanding of diagnosing cancer.

I understand that the 'type' of cancer that they tell you that you have, is only stating where in your body it has shown up. Cancer is systemic, and just because they say that the cancer is______, does not mean that the rest of your body is healthy. You need to heal your body as a whole.

This is where the medical system does a huge disfavor to the public. It gives the false illusion that if they discovered cancer in a certain area, they need to remove it, poison it or radiate it... then you will be okay. They are not addressing the root cause of why you have developed cancer in the first place.

Even though I understand that in reality, cancer is cancer, and that your body is desperate for you to assist it to come back into balance as a whole, I decided to organize this chapter under the labels that these individuals AND YOU were given. I know how it comforts us to read about someone else who had the same 'type' of cancer as we were told that we have.

I want to encourage you to read all of the testimonials, as they all have their own nuggets that you might find helpful, even if they were not labeled the same as you were.

As a disclaimer; each person's testimonial is their own personal experience with their cancer. You will notice that a lot of the things that I discussed earlier in the book, most people also followed either some or all of what I found helpful, before our paths ever crossed. Some chose to do things, that I wouldn't have chosen, but we all need to make our own choices.

Brain Tumor

Julie Tiller

Life changes when you hear that your health is not what it seems.

Back in Jan 2018 I had a cold. Even though the cold left, I still had some weird symptoms. My ears had an echo, like they had to 'pop' and couldn't. At times like they were underwater and ringing. Also, when getting up fast, my eyes would black out for 30 seconds, and then dizzy and black spots... Then the black spots and blurry vision got worse. Not just when I got up too fast, it happened all the time. So, I finally went to the doctor three months later, after my family and friends kept telling me to go.

The doctor thought it was me just being low in my salt and water. Over the next month, nothing got better. They checked my blood pressure and said that I had Orthostatic Hypertension which is when your blood pressure suddenly shoots up when you stand.

As things were not getting any better with my ears, as well as my blacking out, I decided to see a hearing specialist. They assured me that my hearing was fine, so that was not causing the symptoms.

While taking my kids in for their yearly eye tests, I decided to ask the doctor if there was any type of test that he could do, that might give me a clue why my vision would go black all of a sudden.

When he did the test, he found that both my optic nerves were swollen. He immediately got me into see an Eye Surgeon the very next day.

When the Eye Surgeon saw my results, he called the hospital to get me in for a CT scan ASAP. Two days later, they had me in for a CT scan. They found a brain tumor the size of a Canadian Toonie.

My whole sense of life changed. My dreams for the future. My thought patterns, and my whole way of seeing things around me changed, when I saw the tumor on the CT scan.

Quickly they got me in for an MRI. What it showed was that the tumor was attached to a vein. In order to remove it, he would have to cut the tumor apart and scrape it off of the vein, while leaving part of the tumor inside. Then they would start radiation.

Up to this point I had been on the fence about having surgery, as I just wanted to feel better. I didn't understand at the time, the possible ramifications of having surgery. But when I heard that it was attached to a vein, I knew that I did not want to risk the surgery. I also knew that I would not agree to radiation either, as I have always believed that chemotherapy and radiation were not my answer.

My parents and step mom, all encouraged me to listen to God and do what I felt I needed to do. So, after reading parts of the unfinished manuscript of this and her previous book that my step-mom was writing, I bought a juicer and started to juice. I began to work towards eating 80% raw and 20% cooked. I cut out most processed foods and sugar. Now, I still eat some things I shouldn't, but for the most part I'm trying my best. I also understood that major stress had been a huge factor in my developing the tumor. With two young children who love to 'bug' each other, I knew that was going to be a huge hurdle, so I prayed for guidance.

I started where I could by doing a 30-day juice fast. Three months later, I did a 40-day fast. After the 40-day fast, most of my symptoms were gone. It was amazing.

When they did the next MRI, they affirmed that the tumor had not grown at all. When the Eye doctor checked my eyes, he told me that my optic nerves were not as swollen as they were six months earlier. Even though he had wanted me to take a drug to help absorb the spinal fluid, but I hadn't taken, he was amazed that my results were so good. He called me 'a mystery'.

Three months later, after another 30-day juice fast, my only symptom left was that I would black out when I got up too fast.

I feel good health wise, my emotions of course are up and down, with some days hardly remembering that I have a brain tumor, and other days barely being able to get out of bed to face the day, as depression has been something that I have struggled with since I was a teenager.

Every day is so different, but I'm so thankful for the life I do have. The Lord really woke me up to get my health back on track and to rely on Him more. He has given me a wonderful family and friends and a promise that "He's got this!".

Breast Cancer

Keri Lawson Breast Cancer invasive lobular carcinoma estrogen and progesterone positive HER2 negative

My journey started in December 2016. I had been under a lot of stress the previous few years with; developing Lyme's disease, 2 shoulder surgeries, learning 3 new jobs, having my 2 sons have 3 military deployments. (two to Iraq, one to Kosovo), watching my brother take his last breath, my dad having congestive heart failure, and dealing with my mom having Alzheimer's.

I knew that I had something going on for about a year, because my nipple on my left breast was newly inverted and I could see dimpling around a lump.

My family had just lost my little brother after a 7-year battle with colon cancer. I watched him suffer through surgeries, chemo and experimental drugs. I felt that it was just too soon for my family to deal with another issue.

The traveling Mammography van came to our little town so I decided to get it checked out. They saw something and had me go to have it checked out. The lady at the Imaging Center gave me a hug after she did the 2nd mammogram. I then had an ultrasound and an MRI. I didn't even have a doctor to send the results to. I asked a lady that I worked with, who her doctor was and made an appointment to have my results sent to him.

He explained to me that the radiologist was 95% sure that it was cancer. He also told me that by law he had to recommend surgery, chemo and radiation. I told him I didn't plan on doing any of it. He then showed me a list of alternative treatments. I told him I was already doing several things on the list from the research I had been doing on my own.

I had a biopsy in April 2017 and 24 hours after the biopsy I took the little strips off the incision and inserted black salve into the hole. The doctor had concurred with my thought that it would be a direct route to the tumor.

The results came back the following week saying that it was invasive lobular carcinoma estrogen and progesterone positive HER2 negative. I already knew in my heart that it was cancer because it looked just like what I had seen with others with breast cancer.

I salved for 1 1/2 years and supported my immune system by taking sugar out of my diet, eating lots of raw fruits and vegetables, juiced a lot of carrot and celery, ate apricot kernels, took black seed oil, ate hedgeapples, Vit D, Vit C, magnesium. I had all of the metal fillings removed from my mouth, had my elders anoint me with oil and pray over me. I did soul searching to make sure I was not harboring any unforgiveness. I did a lot of rebounding and jumping on the trampoline to move the lymph system. I took long walks in the sunshine, along with doing deep breathing, and coffee enemas. I did a lot of meditating on the Lord's Prayer and the 23rd Psalm.

I would mix it up of what I was doing, thinking that I didn't want the cancer to know what I would hit it with next. I did days of fasting, days of just juice. I didn't eat red meat for at least a year.

When the black salve would be pulling and there was pain, I used clove oil and a heating pad. I didn't take any pain killer because I didn't want anything interfering with my body's ability to heal.

I have learned that the body is an amazing vessel that wants to live, and given the right fuel is able to heal. I know that I have many people that love me, who were worried that I was being foolish. But I was listening to what I felt was the right thing for me. I knew nothing of black salve before I started this journey. I trusted that God would lead the way.

One day when I was feeling low, I went and saw my mom in the Alzheimer's unit in the nursing home. She didn't know who I was at this point, but I told her I had breast cancer and I needed her prayers. She looked right at me, and said "I thought so" and put her head on her hands and cried. It was a gift from God for me to receive, just that one moment of clarity, that I knew my mom understood.

I have learned so much from this journey and as Gilbert K Chesterson once said "A woman uses her intelligence to find reasons to support her intuition!" I am thankful for life and this journey and for all that have had a part!

Stephaney Dunleavy

Grade 2 invasive breast cancer,

estrogen positive, 2cm tumour

I was only 29, when I was diagnosed with breast cancer. I wasn't expecting it to happen to me. Does anyone?

While initially it came as a shock, I was already armed with the understanding that we ourselves are capable of creating our reality based on what we think and the choices we make, so I refused to be crippled by the fear that is associated with cancer.

I knew that I could get better and heal myself, and I vowed to not only survive it, but to thrive in it.

Switching to a vegan diet, juicing and giving my body everything it was seemingly lacking, has definitely helped. But the most crucial part of getting better has been the work I have done on my inner self.

It's been an inside job through and through, and such a journey that it's hard to put into words. I guess the only way to describe it is that cancer made me better.

The choices I made for my healing – i.e. not going down the conventional medicine route, were met with resistance. I had many a meeting with medical professionals who suggested I was making a very bad decision or even that I was crazy. And not all of my family agreed with what I was doing...

While, looking back, I can see that they were coming from a place of care, they were doing so due to their own fears.

Nobody ever achieved anything extraordinary being confined to the limitations of other people. I knew that in order to do this my way, I had to ignore the fears of everyone else. I had to go against the grain.

My refusal to not let anyone influence my decisions or decide my fate, is one of the most rewarding lessons I've gained out of this.

In just under a year from starting my healing journey, my scans have shown that cancer is no longer present in my body, hallelujah!

Jill

Stage 1 Invasive lobular breast cancer

I was diagnosed three years ago. While mine was not very aggressive and I did have surgery, I declined hormone therapy with tamoxifen.

I learned that I could balance my estrogen naturally through diet and lifestyle changes. My protocol is also focused on healing the different key pathways in our body, such as liver detox, lymphatic congestion, gut health and microbiome, circulation and kidneys, brain health etc. My husband was recently diagnosed with aggressive kidney cancer and even conventional medicine acknowledges there is no effective treatment so we are pursuing a holistic approach with him as well.

My diagnosis feels like it was just a primer for the real deal of my husband's diagnosis.

Esther Anderson

Stage 2 Ductal Breast Cancer

I first noticed a dimple in my right breast which became internally hot and cold and occasionally painful. Due to having a younger sister who died the year before, from a very aggressive form of breast cancer at only 47 years old, I was seen very quickly. They diagnosed me with having Ductal Breast Cancer (which is the most common type). I felt a huge relief to know that it wasn't the same type as my sister had.

They told me that it was small and it was not in my underarm. Unfortunately, after 13 mammograms, 10 biopsy's, 3 chest X-rays, an MRI, bone and CT scan, and then performing a mastectomy, it was shown that I had 5 separate lumps as well as it being in my underarm. I was surprised that contrary to all the tests and imaging originally done, it WAS extensive.

Having my breast and lymph nodes removed was what I felt was the best option for me. I believed that it would remove the cancer from my body.

After the mastectomy, I was encouraged to have 15 sessions of radiation, as well as to start taking Tamoxifen.

Even though I live in Scotland, where it is unusual for someone to choose the natural route, I declined both. At the outset I knew I wasn't keen on drugs or treatments, as

I have always preferred to do things naturally. Instead, I wanted to concentrate on diet and homeopathy to minimize the risks of recurrence.

Animals have oestrogen so I have chosen to eat plant based and organic. I have also eliminated sugar as sugar grows tumours. Homeopathic powders have targeted oestrogen regulation. I hope to be cancer free for the rest of my lifetime but, if it should return, I will take responsibility for it. I am not afraid of it. God has given me His peace.

Esophageal and Colon Cancer

Dawn W

Hi my name is Dawn and I am a 2x cancer THRIVER. I was diagnosed with esophageal cancer in 2004 when I was 51. The doctors said it was a man's disease commonly seen in their seventies. I was a rare case being much younger and being a woman. Later I was also told the survival rate was 5%. I refused chemo and radiation so the surgeon said he washed his hands of me and I would have the same cancer back in five years and there was nothing they could do for me. As I write this, it is March 19, 2019 and here I am still esophageal cancer free. In 2017 I was diagnosed with 2 types of colon cancer and a gene carrier of lynch syndrome. I had 4 doctors tell me in order to save my life I needed a complete colon removal, chemo, radiation and wear a colostomy bag the rest of my life. I was 64.

I said no thank you, I would rather have quality of life. One doctor was very scared for me and had his nurse call me several times trying to get me to change my mind and have radical surgery. I finally said give me 3 months to do this my way. She conceded and I did it my way. In April of 2018 it was confirmed I was cancer free.

My story starts back in 1991 when my Dad was diagnosed with colon cancer. The big C word and the fear that is connected with it. Dad had surgery having part of his colon removed. He did awesome.

After that relatives on both sides of my Dad's family came forward saying that they had had colon cancer and they were living quality lives. The only person who had died of colon cancer at that point was my Dad's Mom when my Dad was 18 which would have been in the early 40's. A few years later Dad was diagnosed with Prostate cancer, he was given radiation. My sister was diagnosed with Uterine cancer, she was given radiation. My active sister became disabled, my Dad was no longer as energetic. My brother was diagnosed with colon cancer. My Dad was then diagnosed with Lymphoma, the chemo treatments started and his quality of life went downhill. My sister was then diagnosed with colon cancer and her chemo treatments began. She beat colon cancer but she could no longer work because her energy levels would come in spurts and then she would be in bed for days or more. She also developed skin cancer.

I was a Cosmetologist and became interested in the "Look Good Feel Better" program helping cancer patients learn how to make themselves feel good through make up, scarves, turbines and wigs. I shaved many heads and fitted them to wigs. So, I was seeing firsthand what chemo and radiation was doing to people's quality of life. I went to several funerals of clients because they lost their battle.

I had a Christian friend ask me to help her through another battle with cancer. She had started with uterine cancer, skin cancer, then colon cancer. She had surgeries and chemo. Now the cancer had gone into her liver, she had several tumors, with one being the size of an orange. We were involved in a ministry that teaches about Biblical healings. I took a reference page out of the syllabus and we prayed and went over every account of that page. Daily I was building the Word of God into my heart and mind. This went on for months so the Word was established in me. Her tumor had shrunk, so she went for surgery to remove them. She made it and was put on more chemo.

Then I wasn't feeling well. I thought I was out of shape so I started a kick boxing class. Instead of getting energized I became weaker, I was having trouble swallowing. The doctor told me to chew my food better.

From March until October I was telling this doctor there was something wrong with me and he didn't listen until I told him I can't even swallow water. I already had a colostomy appointment just because of the family history so an endoscopy was tagged on to it.

I prayed that the procedures would show what the problem was so it could be addressed. We were thinking I would have to have my esophagus stretched.

The doctor said, "I must have had my eyeballs on good today because I found an ulcerated area under the flap where the stomach and esophagus meet." I was put on medication to try to heal it because they thought it was probably caused by the stomach acid.

Well, it wasn't. I went to the doctors alone and was told, "You have esophageal cancer and it has been growing for about 3 years." I started to cry and then said to myself, wait a minute. I have all this Word of God in me. I can't cry I just have to claim what I know.

I went home, told my husband and we made a plan to be positive and do whatever we had to glorify God. II Timothy 1:7 was my verse; "God did not give me the spirit of fear but of power love and a sound mind." I went forward believing this was a process I had to do to get the cancer out of me and I would be fine. I was positive. I allowed no negative people around me.

Surgery was December 17, 2004. I was in the ICU the shortest amount anyone with this surgery ever was. I had things done to me that no one should ever go through but I stayed my mind on God and His healing power. They cut me from shoulder blade to belly button. They cut vertically the length of the left side of my neck where they pulled the diseased part out through. They cut out 1/3 of my stomach and my esophagus up to behind my heart. They cut my sternum to pull my left ribcage out of the way. They held my arm in a position to keep it out of the way over extending which later caused me to have rotator cuff surgery. They pulled my remainder stomach up to meet what was left of my esophagus and stapled them together wrapping a wire around the tube they just made to hold it in place. Forty-seven lymph nodes were also removed. Then they glued me back together.

After a period. I was sent to rehab to be fitted to a feeding tube. After that was done, I went home where I was cared for round the clock and had in-home nurses. There were some bumps in the healing road that were rough but we got through them. I finally was taken off the feeding tube a few months later.

Three different oncologists said there was something unusual about my body because when they did the biopsy, the size of the cancer was smaller. When they did the biopsy on the 47 lymph nodes they could not find any cancer where it had been. I looked at them and said "God Healed Me" they said God had nothing to do with it, you have a unique body and we want to do chemo and radiation on you because you probably have more cancer in you. Your insurance won't pay for this cocktail we want to do, it will burn out your esophagus and your lungs. I asked them if they were even listening to what they were saying. No, I'm not doing that.

By the time I got to the surgeon's office he had heard and was furious with me and told me the cancer would be back in 5 years and there was nothing they could do for me. I went out of there upset and also knowing he was not God and if I was blowing their minds with the way I was recovering God would continue to work in me to not get it again.

That started my holistic search besides the foods they wanted me to eat after I got the feeding tube out almost killed me.

I found Chris Wark, he was diagnosed the same year as me. I bought a Jack Lalane juicer and started juicing. I continued to search for answers as to why my family was so riddled with cancer.

I learned about pH balance and became certified as a coach. I learned how to alkalize my system. Because of the trauma my body went through, a few things happened. My body went into Graves disease and I almost died, but was put on medication.

A few years later my body started acting like I was having another Graves episode. A specialist in Cardiology discovered the Vegas nerve to my heart had been cut. This is the main nerve and also plays a major role in digestion. He said I'm sorry I can't fix you. I was put on more medication. I said; "that's ok because God can heal me."

Meanwhile my sister was diagnosed with pancreatic cancer, my Dad was still going back and forth with lymphoma. The treatments were destroying his stomach. He was having to have blood transfusions every couple of months, because they found he was bleeding internally. He had to have his stomach cauterized several times.

I told my sister WHEN you beat the pancreatic cancer, I will take you to the Bahamas. I didn't even have a job!

It worked out that I took her to the Bahama's, and that was the last time I would take a trip with my little sister.

While I was studying about nutrition, detoxing, pH balance, essential oils, supplements, herbs and different holistic cancer treatments and searching for what was best for me to live, my Dad, my little sister and my best friend were all dying listening to conventional medicine.

When I was at my friends who had a 50% survival rate, her treatment was delivered in a hazmat package. I read the instructions, do not touch with your fingers or your lips but take it internally. WHAT!!!! Are you kidding? I asked how she takes it and is this really what you want to do. I watched as she poured a pill into the lid of the container, tipped her head back and dropped it into the back of her throat and swallowed.

She died a couple of years later because I believe that chemo treatment ate up her insides. My Dad died in 2009 having had 4 different cancers, my little sister died in 2013 having had 6 different cancers, my best friend died in 2014.

My Dad didn't want to change how he ate, I didn't push. My sister tried to eat better and she researched along with me but the damage was so extensive that the doctors even admitted that she had had too much radiation and chemo previously and her body couldn't handle it. She weighed about 87 pounds when she took her last breath while I was holding her hand. My friend ate very well when I was taking care of her and she tried but well-meaning friends who could not understand nutrition kept bringing her comfort food to cheer her up. How could she say no? My friend died with her high school friends around her in 2014. Can anyone understand why I refused chemo and radiation when I saw so many lose quality of life from it?

I was able to go back to work and got so much energy that one day while at our family camp, I out hiked two teenage boys up the hill through the woods. I was so proud.

Life went on and I was doing very well. Then where I worked closed, so I was out of a job. We had to move. Many negative things hit at once, along with people saying you are fine now, have some ice cream, have some candy and I started eating badly. It doesn't take long to pick up bad habits along with carrying much stress.

I started to not feel well. I was due for an endoscopy and colonoscopy, and in August of 2017, I was diagnosed with 2 types of colon cancer and a couple of other polyps.

They wanted to cut me up. I said, "I listened to you before, you have sliced and diced me and as a result I went into Graves, you cut my Vegas nerve and I had to have rotator cuff surgery besides which I was in pain for 3 years because my rib cage was not put back in place and a chiropractor had to fix that." Now four doctors want to save my life by taking my whole colon and I wear a colostomy bag. I could live with a colostomy bag if I had to. My best friend had one and I learned to clean hers so I knew the procedure and I knew the daily concerns of it. The point is, if I had to.

I was searching for a functional doctor to go to. The Cleveland Clinic had a waiting list of a year. I don't have time for that. The doctors were calling; the chemo treatments are different now. You need to do this. They wanted to save my life. They wanted to save my life in 2004 and I am still recovering from that. They wanted to save my Dad's life, my sister's, my best friend. They are all gone and I miss them terribly.

God is bigger and greater than anything man can do. Psalms 103:3 says; "Who forgives all your iniquities; who heals all diseases." He said ALL diseases. God designed the body to heal itself.

Cancer I have learned is a symptom that the immune system has been compromised. God says in His Word that He will supply ALL of our need. So, who am I going to listen to? God provided the herbs of the earth to be eaten.

In July, I had looked in our yard and said "wow, we have a lot of dandelions this year." In August after I was diagnosed, I said, "thank you God for supplying my way to be healed with all these dandelions." We went out and dug up the dandelions, we made powder from the roots. Dandelions were eaten at every meal. Powder sprinkled on meals, into teas, the greens in my morning egg, in my salads, in every vegetable I ate. God supplied me with dandelions for my liver and blood to be cleansed.

I wrote up my own health plan with all the information I had been absorbing for years. I made a plan and stuck with it. I eventually found a functional chiropractor who set up reasonable payment plans. He was impressed with my plan and said he wouldn't change anything. I received adjustments, micro current, foot detox, vibration board and oxygen and they did a complete bloodwork panel. I did a 12-week program for candida. I was so thankful I was led to this wellness center. They were all believers so healing started taking place the second you stepped through the doors. They were all positive, Biblical based quotes were around the office. I could listen to healing scriptures on a headset while getting micro current.

My husband had purchased an infrared sauna which I used regularly besides doing coffee enemas, and many other things to build my immune system so my body would heal itself.

In April 2018 with bloodwork proof it was confirmed that I was cancer free. I did it my way, which was how God worked in me without surgery, chemo, radiation and I don't wear a colostomy bag. As a bonus I came off all conventional medications and no longer need the specialists.

I share my story believing someone may be inspired to know that our God is greater than anything the world may throw our way. Greater is He that is in you than he that is in the world. God's abounding blessings for healing and prosperity.

Lung Cancer

Janine Gundert

Stage 3b Lung Cancer

Being diagnosed with stage 3b lung cancer in October of 2015 felt like being dropped from the top of a fifty storey building. There I was, splat on the pavement, unable to move, frozen it seemed. Frozen in fear and paralyzed by anxiety.

As a self-confessed control freak, it was a horrible aha moment of "you are so not in control right now". That was the time that I lost my emotional footing, dropped to my knees, and placed the whole "c" thing at God's feet. I knew this was something I could not battle alone.

Where to start? What to do? How to control the fear that kept me from moving. Prayer brought me what I asked for. The cloak of God's peace covered me and allowed me to start moving. It opened up my mind and heart to receive the ideas and the direction I needed to make decisions about what treatment options I was comfortable with.

I was led by God to a Christian hospital in Mexico that has been treating cancer patients for over fifty years. They use integrated therapies (some main stream medical) and many natural treatments.

Between November of 2015 and February of 2018, I was under their care and had many treatments such as; hyperthermia, ozonated oxygen, high dose vitamin C infusions, dendritic cell vaccine, complete lifestyle change including diet and emotional healing. I was also taking a targeted drug for a gene mutation identified in the cancer I was diagnosed with.

I was blessed to be in remission from May to November of 2017, but unfortunately that did not last. I experienced disease progression on my next two scans so I knew I had to change something.

During that time, I had connected with a beautiful soul through Facebook and she had healed her body of breast cancer almost four years previous and had been cancer free ever since. I connected with her spiritually (she too has a strong connection to our creator) and emotionally. She is very knowledgeable about the protocol she had used so I followed her lead.

I have been doing the Cellect protocol since March of last year. One thing I have learned through experience, is that my body has a very low tolerance for drugs. This protocol is natural.

I currently do not take any drugs. I continue with the lifestyle changes I have made and will not go back. That old way of living is what brought this to me in the first place! I eat organic produce most of the time and have greatly reduced my intake of animal protein and dairy. In addition, I have eliminated sugar. I don't eat any canned or processed goods and I drink reverse osmosis filtered water. I have replaced household cleaners and personal care items with natural versions (no chemicals), in other words, I have assessed everything that I put into my body, and onto my body, top to bottom and have cleaned house!

As well as giving my body what it needs to heal physically, I feed my mind with positivity and God's word. When I give my mind the right material to work with, it helps to keep my emotions from running my day, running my life.

For years I was highly stressed, full of resentment and bitterness that I clung too. I became comfortable with being that way and didn't know how to let go. Thankfully, through a lot of personal development (courses and reading in particular) I realized that my negative feelings were not only hurting others who I love, but myself as well. I needed to love ME more! Letting go of all that negativity was a huge step forward and it freed my mental and emotional energy to improve my life in other ways.

Learning to set boundaries in my life and to acknowledge who I am and what works for me in my life were ways I could love myself as well. I am much calmer, happier and content than I have ever been. I realize now that the mental and emotional healing that we need to do is just as important as the physical healing. And I'm confident that I'm headed in the right direction and will one day be cancer free.

My scan of August 2018 showed that the disease was at the very least "controlled". My most recent scan shows improvements (yay!). So I just need to continue doing what I am doing, putting one foot in front of the other, taking it day by day, and allowing God to lead me where he wants me to go.

Throughout this healing journey, I have seldom felt overwhelmed. It has felt as if God places a stepping stone in my path and directs me to it, and then he shows me the next step. No getting ahead of myself there! And a good reminder that I am still not in control. But the peace he has brought me throughout this journey allows me to be okay with that. I believe that my body will eventually heal itself. God created our bodies to heal. We just need to give them what they need in order to do that. We are wondrously made. I'm learning to respect that and to appreciate that. Life is so wonderful! And God is amazing!

Testicular Cancer

Geoff Waterman
Bilateral Testicular Cancer /
Stage 3 Neuroendocrine Cancer

In 2012 I was diagnosed with Stage 1 Non- Seminoma Testicular Cancer. Before I even had time to process the diagnoses, they had me in for an Orchiectomy (removal of a testis). Three weeks later, my urologist wanted me to have another ultrasound. I was then re-diagnosed as "Bilateral" Testicular Cancer and they wanted to do surgery immediately to remove the other testis.

I was directed to do radiation and/or chemotherapy. Not knowing anything about cancer, I followed what the doctors were telling me, and went for a consultation with the radiologist. I then had a second consultation with an oncologist who instructed me on the "benefits" of doing chemotherapy. I decided on chemotherapy and completed one round 2 weeks later.

I became so sick within 12 hours of finishing my infusion, that I had to return to the Cancer Center and spent the whole day there till they could get all my issues under control. Three weeks later, I went back to do my 2nd treatment, but when I walked into the room, I had a strong feeling that this was not a good idea, so I left vowing to not do anymore chemotherapy. (I would later realize that strong feeling was God warning me not to do it)

Fast forward 4 years, January 2017, I was at, what I thought, would be my final oncology appointment. I was excited that I would never have to return to the Cancer Center again. I was going to celebrate with a huge banana split. Little did I know, that I was about to hit a brick wall.

As I was getting my coat on to leave, the nurse turned the computer screen toward me with the results of my CT Scan. It stated that they had found two tumors in my small intestines. It appeared to be Neuroendocrine Carcinoid Cancer. I was floored!

I was sitting there in a daze as she was explaining everything to me, wondering to myself how this could happen. I had followed all of their protocols for follow up, bloodwork and scans so how could this happen?

At the end of the appointment she handed me a pile of paperwork with all of these new appointments that were already made for me. I was booked for appointments for scans, oncologist, surgeon as well as a cardiologist since they had to check my heart to make sure the cancer did not affect my heart, which this type of cancer does deteriorate the valves. It was all just a blur but yet they had taken care of everything for me, or did they?

I had believed them over the last four years, when they told me that what they had done had worked. Here I had started with Stage 1 Bilateral" Testicular Cancer, and now they were telling me that I had developed Stage 3 Neuroendocrine Cancer!

About 7 weeks later I had the surgery. While in my hospital room the nurse came in with a regular food menu. I looked it over and told her I thought there was a mistake. I told her that this couldn't be right. This was not the type of food I expected to eat after they just removed part of my small intestines and 23 lymph nodes.

She returned 30 mins. later and stated that the doctor said there were NO dietary restrictions. What?? NO restrictions?? This was my wake-up call! The medical System was no longer making sense to me.

I knew that I had to find answers that made more sense. I started researching, and found a vast amount of other people who were treating their cancer by doing things that made more rational sense. I learned that I shouldn't be eating sugar, dairy or red meat, as they feed cancer. I watched the video series "The Truth About Cancer". I started reading what "Chris Wark Beat Cancer" was sharing, I found "Cancer Tutor". I researched which foods were the most helpful, as well as juicing protocols.

About a month later, I had changed my diet to a NO sugar, no red meat, mostly plant-based diet. Every morning for breakfast, I juiced about 30 oz of carrots, celery, a small beet, a small piece of ginger and a green apple. Of course, these are all organic. I then added in; lemon juice and Braggs Apple Cider Vinegar, as well as the powders of organic Amla, Moringa, and greens, I do essential oils of frankincense, lavender and lemon daily. We rid our home of toxic cleaners and bought a Berkey water system. I also drink Sir Jason Winters tea and dandelion root tea daily.

I started seeing a naturopath. I immediately did a curcumin protocol and continue to take curcumin daily. I did oxygen therapy. I take apricot seeds, mushroom supplements, vitamin C and vitamin D3.

The most important thing out of all of this, is I repaired my relationship with my Lord and Savior Jesus Christ. I don't believe that I would be still alive, if it weren't for Him. God did not give me cancer. He may have allowed it to happen, but if He didn't use it to help me put my trust in Him, instead of the doctors, I would hate to think of where I'd be now without Him. He pointed me in the right direction and showed me how He made our bodies to heal naturally with what He has provided for us.

I truly believe subjecting my body to the toxins of chemotherapy, weakened my immune system even more than it already was. I have since discovered that surgery opens the gates for cancer to spread to other parts of my body, which it did. I also believe that the reason I am in my second year of remission from Stage 3 Neuroendocrine Cancer is, from getting my relationship right with God. I thank God for every day that I have and continue to learn and share how natural and holistic living can change your life. I am now 65 lbs lighter and so much healthier than I was 7 years ago at the age of 44.

Advanced Uterine Cancer

Veronica Ivonne

Full recovery after been given less than two weeks to live

October 2011, I went in to the emergency room because I was in severe pain. I had not urinated in two days. I had a large tumor, which I was unaware of, blocking my bladder.

After clearing my bladder with a catheter, they did a bunch of tests, and told me I had advanced uterine cancer, and that I needed a hysterectomy and chemo.

I refused chemo after I was told I had less than 2 weeks to live. I was told chemo would add an additional 2 years. I said "No thank you." I told them that they may remove only part of my tumor without touching any of my organs.

The doctors in the hospital told me that I was crazy. They shook their heads and frowned. They called in a psychiatrist to evaluate me. I passed the evaluation. Then they called in another psychiatrist and I passed the second evaluation.

I told the doctors that I would sue if I left the hospital without my organs. They wanted me to sign forms but I refused to sign anything. I gave them verbal permission to remove only part of my tumor and nothing else.

After I left the hospital, I went to Hippocrates Health Institute for two months. There I followed the Hippocrates diet and drank 6 glasses of green juice everyday for the two months that I was there.

When I returned to New York City, I went to see an oncologist and gynecologist. My cancer was almost cleared. I continued on Hippocrates Diet for the rest of the year. I went to the oncologist again and told I was cleared. My cancer cleared within a year. I've been cancer-free since 2012.

If you have cancer or a history of cancer STOP eating meat, chicken, pork, eggs, milk, cheese, yogurt and all other forms of animal fat/protein!

My current diet:
50% raw fruits, 50% raw veggies (roots, tomatoes, bell peppers and leafy greens). Nothing from a can, bottle, or box. The main importance to ridding my cancer was being on 100% raw plant diet.

Disclaimer:
Any information contained in this post is strictly for educational purposes. It does not involve the diagnosing, treatment, or prescribing of remedies for the treatment of diseases.

Where to Go from Here

We are now coming to a close of our time together. I really hope that if you have not already gotten started on rebuilding your health, that you will start now. You can have awesome energy and a body that heals itself, it just takes a burning desire, and determination to become healthier than you have been in years. It will take making changes. You CAN do it!

I know that sometimes it may feel like you are on this health rebuilding journey all by yourself. You don't want to stress out your loved ones, with all of the different emotions and thoughts that you are struggling with.

If they are not in agreement with your decision to reject the medical model, and go the natural route instead, you do not want to give them any reason to start pressuring you to "give up this foolishness". Besides, you sense that they are having their own challenges attempting to stay strong for you.

Then there are your friends. They are great, but maybe they haven't had this type of experience, so you don't believe that they can truly understand what you are going through; the fears, the doubts, the regrets, and coming face to face with the prospect of dying.

I remember when I was pregnant with my first child. Even though I was engaged to be married when I discovered that I was pregnant, I went through a range of emotions. Unfortunately, I confided in my doctor what I was thinking, and feeling. I expected to receive some affirming words to tell me that what I was feeling was normal, and that everything would be okay.

What I received instead was a strong rebuke from this doctor. He told me that if I was feeling these feelings, that I would be a horrible mother. I definitely had chosen the wrong person to seek comfort from. Needless to say, I started searching for a new doctor immediately... once I stopped crying.

Feeling discouraged is a very real emotion that some of us go through. The last thing you need is to be confronted with someone who has no clue of what you are going through, when you are barely holding on emotionally yourself.

We need others to direct us back to the truth, rather than listening to the lies of the enemy. For this important reason, I will be offering an online program that will support both you as well as your loved ones on this journey called 'Goodbye Cancer, Hello Health'.

It will give you the opportunity to be surrounded by others who totally understand what you are going through, because they have also experienced cancer. Besides additional education, and support on following all of the health principals that was discussed earlier, you will find yourself in a private online group where you can hang out, be real with what you are thinking or feeling, ask questions, get support, give support, and not stress out your family and friends when "You just need to talk about what is going through your mind."

Your loved one, can also be supported in a separate private group, where they can talk freely about what they are going through, again without adding to what you are emotionally dealing with.

If you would like to work further with me, and this sounds like something that you are interested in finding out more about, then head on over to www.GoodbyeCancerHelloHealth.com to get more information.

If you have received everything that you need for now, WONDERFUL! Love to hear about your healing journey. Drop me a quick note through Messenger to say "hi". My Facebook and Messenger account is under 'Donna Marie Hockley'.

In the meantime, I would like to leave you with Psalms 103:2 – 4

"Bless the Lord, O my soul,
And forget not all His benefits:
Who forgives all your iniquities,
Who heals all your diseases,
Who redeems your life from destruction,
Who crowns you with loving kindness
and tender mercies."

Chat soon ☺
Donna Marie Hockley

Made in the USA
Monee, IL
25 January 2021